Sex Education Dictionary

Sex
Education
Dictionary

Gill Mullinar

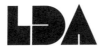

Based on the original US edition
by Dr Dean Hoch and Nancy Hoch

To John, Timothy and Nicholas, with love.

Acknowledgements

I would like to thank my editor, Sheila White, for her patience, hard work and friendship; Hounslow and Spelthorne Health Education Unit for their help and support; Dr Michael Purves for his extremely helpful comments, often given at short notice; Dr J Newman; Julie and Aleine; Nicola, Portia and my parents for their help with childcare at desperate moments; and the rest of my family who kept me going throughout the writing of this book.

Sex Education Dictionary
Edited by Sheila White
Designed by John Wright
Illustrated by David Gifford
Cover cartoons by Jon Riley
Photoset by Domino Typesetting

LD643
ISBN 1 85503 138 8
© text Gill Mullinar
© illustrations David Gifford
© cover cartoons Jon Riley
All rights reserved
First published 1992

LDA
Duke Street, Wisbech
Cambridgeshire PE13 2AE
England

Contents

To young people everywhere   7

How to use this dictionary   9

Definitions   11

Drawings of male and
    female anatomy   114-115

To parents, carers and anyone
    working with young people   116

To teachers   118

Useful addresses   119

To young people everywhere

The **Sex Education Dictionary** is for you. It contains definitions of words which are to do with sex, personal relationships and pregnancy and birth.

Most of us have a natural interest in how our bodies and feelings change as we grow older. But many people find it difficult to talk openly about relationships and sex. This can be a problem if you read or hear a word and you don't know what it means or if you want to find out more about something and there's no-one to ask. Many words to do with sex and personal relationships aren't in ordinary dictionaries. Even if you do find a word in an ordinary dictionary, the explanation might be too difficult to understand and leave you just as confused.

So this dictionary has been written for you to use on your own or to share with others. It won't teach you everything there is to know about sex. But it should:

- help you to find out or check the meaning of over 350 words and terms to do with personal relationships, sex, pregnancy and birth
- give you information about how your body changes as you grow older and about the many different ways in which people express themselves sexually
- make it clear to you that you have rights over your own body and feelings and that you can make choices
- help put your mind at rest if you have any worries about your own growth and development
- help you become more aware of the different opinions and beliefs people have about sex and about what is – and what isn't – acceptable and responsible behaviour

● help you to tell the difference between slang words, which can shock and offend people, and words which are okay to use with a parent, teacher, doctor or other adult.

The definitions are straightforward and easy to understand. But you might find that sometimes a definition contains a difficult word which stops you understanding the rest of the definition. If this happens, ask someone to help you. They might be able to tell you what the difficult word means or they might know how you can find out.

One final word. Before you look up anything in the dictionary, please read the next section, **How to use this dictionary**. It won't take you long to read it and it should help you get a lot more out of the dictionary.

How to use this dictionary

Here is an example of a definition from the **Sex Education Dictionary**. The notes should help you get more out of the definitions.

You can find a drawing of the fallopian tubes on page 115.

This is how you say (or pronounce) the word 'fallopian'. 'LO' is in capital letters because it is the part of the word which you emphasise. So 'fallopian' has this rhythm – di-<u>dar</u>-di-di (fa-LO-pee-an).

If there is a group of words in italics (like *this*), start by looking up the first word if you need to (in this case under 'f' for 'female'). If

that doesn't tell you all you want to know, look up the next word too (in this case under 'r' for 'reproductive system').

fallopian tube (fa-LO-pee-an) Part of the *female reproductive system* . There are two fallopian tubes (see the drawing on page 115). They are muscular tubes, one on each side of the *uterus* . Every month as part of the *menstrual cycle*, an ovum is released by one *ovary* into the fallopian tube nearest to it (see *ovulation*) . If a woman has *sexual intercourse* with a man around this time, the ovum may be fertilised by a *sperm* in the fallopian tube. See *fertilisation* and *ectopic pregnancy.*

A word which you can look up in this dictionary is only in italics (like *this*) the <u>first time</u> it appears in a definition.

The words 'woman' and 'man' (not 'girl' or 'boy') are used in this dictionary when the definition is referring to sexual activity.

This means that you can find more information by looking up 'ovulation' in this dictionary.

A word in italics (like *this*) is in this dictionary and you can look it up (in this case under 'u' because 'uterus' starts with a 'u').

A

abdomen (AB-der-mun) The part of the body between the chest and the top of the legs which contains *organs* such as the stomach, the liver and the intestines. In a girl or woman, the *uterus* is in the abdomen.

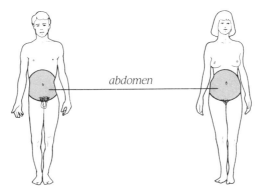

abdomen

abortion (a-BOR-shun) The ending of a *pregnancy*. This can either be a spontaneous abortion (see *miscarriage*) or when a pregnancy is ended on purpose by removing the *embryo* or *fetus* from a woman's *uterus*. People have different views about abortion. Some people believe that abortion is wrong because the unborn child has a right to life. Other people believe that abortion is right because a woman should be able to choose whether or not to have the baby. If you are *pregnant* and you are unsure about it, you can get help from one of the organisations listed on pages 119 and 120. The law says that a woman cannot have an abortion if she is more than 24 weeks pregnant unless there is a serious risk to her life or to the baby's life. So if you are pregnant and don't want to be, you need to make sure you get help early in the pregnancy.

abstinence (AB-sti-nens) Abstaining from or not doing something. Can be used to mean choosing not to be involved in *sexual activity* of any kind.

A

abuse See *sexual abuse.*

AC/DC You may find that some people don't like this word. It means *bisexual.*

acne (AK-ni) See *spots.* If you have lots of spots and they are infected and pus-filled, you may have acne. Go to your doctor. She or he may give you two medicines – a cream to open up the pores and an antibiotic for the infection.

Acquired Immune Deficiency Syndrome See *AIDS.*

Adam's apple The bump which sticks out from your throat where your voice box (or larynx) is. As your body grows, your voice box gets bigger too and makes your voice become deeper. Men have larger voice boxes than women so their Adam's apple usually sticks out more and their voices are usually deeper. See *voice changes.*

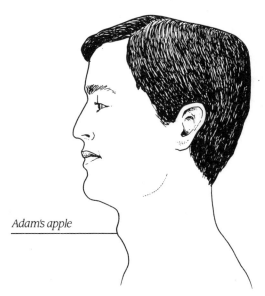

Adam's apple

adolescence (ad-o-LESS-ens) The time of life when a girl changes into a young woman and a boy changes into a young man. Your body changes first (see *puberty*). But during adolescence, you have to grow up *emotionally* too. Sorting out your feelings is not something which happens overnight and being an adolescent can be exciting, confusing, scary or all of these at once! Finding someone you can talk to and share your worries with may help if you find that things are getting you down.

adolescent (ad-o-LESS-ent) Someone who is going through *adolescence*.

adoption (a-DOP-shun) Becoming a permanent member of a new family. You may be adopted if your birth parents die, or if for some unavoidable reason they have had to make the difficult decision to give up their rights to you. Your new family are now your legal parents. You have a new birth certificate so that you share your new family's name. As an adopted child, you have the same rights and status as any other children in the family. You are probably very special to your new family – after all, they chose you! But at some point in your life you may want to find out more about your birth parents. You can get more information about how to do this from the British Agencies for Adoption and Fostering (BAAF). Their address is on page 119.

If you are *pregnant* and cannot keep your baby for some reason, you can ask to have it adopted. But you must talk this through very carefully with someone before you decide. The BAAF and other organisations listed on pages 119 and 120 can help.

adultery (a-DUL-ter-ri) *Sexual intercourse* between two people if one or both of them is married to someone else.

afterbirth The *placenta*, empty *amniotic sac* and *umbilical cord* which together are gently pulled through the woman's *vagina* after her baby has been born.

age of consent Consent means agreeing to something. The age of consent is the age at which the law says a girl can have *sexual intercourse*. In England, Wales and Scotland the age of consent is 16. In Northern Ireland it is 17 and in Eire it is 18. The law assumes that boys under 14 are not capable of having sexual intercourse. A man or boy aged 14 or over commits a crime if he has sexual intercourse with a girl who is under the age of consent. (It does not make any difference if the girl agreed to have intercourse with him – he has still committed a crime.) The girl in this situation is not committing a crime. A girl over the age of consent who has sexual intercourse with a boy under 16 is not breaking the law but she could be charged with indecent assault.

AID Stands for *artificial insemination* by donor.

AIDS Stands for Acquired Immune Deficiency Syndrome. If you have AIDS, your body's *immune system* breaks down so that it

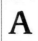

cannot fight off infections. AIDS is caused by a virus called *HIV.* You cannot catch AIDS but you can be infected with HIV. Experts think that most people with HIV eventually get HIV-related symptoms or AIDS. At present there is no cure for AIDS. If you are worried about AIDS or HIV, you can telephone the National AIDS Helpline (their telephone number is on page 120). See *HIV.*

AIDS test See *HIV antibody test.*

AIDS virus Some people use this when they mean *HIV* (the virus which can lead to *AIDS*).

amenorrhoea (a-men-er-REE-a) The absence of *menstruation.* Your *menstrual periods* stop while you are *pregnant.* They might also stop if you are anorexic or if your body's rhythms are disturbed in other ways, for example, after a hospital operation, a bad shock or jet lag.

amniocentesis (am-nee-o-sen-TEE-sis) A test in which a sample of *amniotic fluid* is taken from a *pregnant* woman. This fluid contains some of the unborn baby's *cells.* The results of the test can show up problems with the baby.

amniotic fluid (am-nee-OT-ik) The watery liquid inside the *amniotic sac* (see the drawing on page 72). Also called liquor. The *fetus* floats in this liquid while it develops in the *uterus* during *pregnancy.* Amniotic fluid protects the fetus from bumps and knocks, helps keep its temperature steady and allows it to grow and move around freely. Before or during *labour,* the sac breaks and the fluid drains out from the woman's *vagina.* This is called the waters breaking.

amniotic sac (am-nee-OT-ik) The thin membrane which forms a closed bag around the *fetus* while it is developing in the *uterus* during *pregnancy.* Also called the caul or membrane. The amniotic sac contains the *amniotic fluid.*

anal intercourse (AY-nul) *Sexual intercourse* when a man puts his *penis* through another person's *anus* and into their *rectum.* If two men are having a *sexual relationship* they might decide to have anal intercourse. This is legal (except in Eire, the Isle of Man and Jersey) as long as it is in private and both men are over 21. But if someone who is *HIV*-infected has anal intercourse with you without using a *condom,* there is a high risk of him passing on the virus to you (see *HIV*). This is why many *gay* men now have *safer*

14

sex. Although it is physically possible for a man and a woman to have anal intercourse, it is against the law.

antenatal (an-ti-NAY-tul) Before the *birth* of a baby.

antenatal care (an-ti-NAY-tul) Healthcare of a *pregnant* woman by her doctor and *midwife* to make sure that she and her unborn baby stay fit and well. Once *pregnancy* has been confirmed by a doctor, a woman should have regular *antenatal* check-ups right up to the baby's *birth*.

antibody (AN-ti-bo-di) A protein which the body produces to fight off bacteria or viruses. Antibodies are in our blood. *HIV* invades and kills the blood cells which produce antibodies, leaving the HIV-infected person less able to fight off infections.

anus (AY-nus) The hole at the end of your back passage or *rectum* (see the drawings on pages 114 and 115). When you go to the toilet, *faeces* come out of this hole.

aphrodisiac (af-ro-DI-zee-ak) A substance which is supposed to make you feel more *sexy*. There is no proof that any substance can do this.

areola (a-ree-O-la) On the *breast*, the area of skin which surrounds the *nipple* (see the drawing on page 18). A few stray hairs often grow on the areola.

arousal See *sexual arousal*.

arse This word may shock or offend some people. It means *bottom*. It is also spelt 'ass'.

arsehole This word may shock or offend some people. It means *anus*. It is also spelt 'asshole'.

artificial insemination (ar-ti-FI-shul in-sem-i-NAY-shun) Introducing a man's *sperm* into a woman's *vagina* artificially. Sometimes a man and a woman want a baby but despite regular *sexual intercourse*, the woman does not *conceive*. Or a woman might want a baby but cannot have, or has decided not to have, sexual intercourse with a man. Artificial insemination involves getting the sperm as close as possible to the woman's *cervix* to give it the best chance of entering the *uterus*, meeting an *ovum* and starting a baby (see *fertilisation*).

assertive (a-SER-tiv) If you are assertive, you are firm about what you want and feel but also aware of other people's needs and feelings. Being assertive can be important in a *relationship*, if, for example, you want to say no to *sexual intercourse*, or if you want your *partner* to use a *condom* because you are worried about getting *pregnant* or becoming infected with *HIV.*

B

baby blues Feeling run down and depressed just after having a baby. Baby blues can be caused by tiredness, changing *hormone* levels, sore stitches from the *birth*, sore *breasts* or problems looking after or loving the new baby. The baby blues usually only last a few days. A few women become very depressed (see *postnatal depression*).

back passage Some people use this to mean *rectum.*

balls This word may shock or offend some people. It means *testes.*

barrier method A method of *contraception* which acts as a physical barrier to *sperm*, stopping them from making contact with an *ovum*. Examples are the *diaphragm* and the *condom*. Some barrier methods can also protect against *sexually transmitted infections.*

belly button Some people use this to mean *navel.*

bigamy (BIG-a-mi) Being married to two people at the same time. Bigamy is against the law in the UK.

birth The moment when a baby is born. See *labour.*

birth canal Some people use this to mean *vagina.*

birth control Some people use this to mean *contraception.*

bisexual (by-SEX-you-ul) A word used to describe someone who is sexually attracted to both men and women.

bladder (BLA-der) The sac in the body where *urine* is stored (see the drawings on pages 114 and 115).

blow job This expression may shock or offend some people. It means *fellatio.* See *oral sex.*

blue movie Some people use this to mean a pornographic film. See *pornography.*

BO Stands for body odour. A person who has BO smells unpleasant. After *puberty,* you may sweat more and the area under your arms and between your legs can start to smell if you don't wash regularly. Some *body fluids* such as *urine, vaginal fluid, menstrual blood* and *semen* are clean when they leave the body but once outside it they may also become smelly. To avoid BO, wash, shower or have a bath every day if you can and change your clothes regularly, especially underwear.

body fluids Any fluids which are naturally present in the body such as *semen, vaginal fluid,* blood, *urine,* saliva and so on.

body hair See *hair.*

· **body odour** See *BO.*

bollocks This word may shock or offend some people. It means *testes.*

bondage *Sex* in which one person is tied up and therefore has to do what the other one wants. Most people do not enjoy sex in this way.

boob You may find that some people don't like this word. It means *breast.*

bosom (BUZ-em) Some people use this word instead of *breast.*

bottom The part of your body that you sit on.

bra (BRAR) Underwear for girls and women which covers and supports their *breasts.* If you buy a bra you need to give your *chest* size (eg 30in/65cm, 32in/70cm, 34in/75cm, 36in/80cm) and your cup size (eg AA, A, B, C, D, DD). To get a rough idea of your chest size, first measure yourself right round underneath your breasts, holding the tape measure firmly. Then add 5 inches (12cm) to this measurement. This is your chest size. For your cup size, measure around your breasts where they are largest. If this measurement is 1 inch (2.5cm) less than your chest size, you are an AA cup. If it is the same, you are an A cup. If it is 1 inch more, you are a B cup, and so on. If you are not sure how to measure yourself, you can ask an assistant in the underwear department of a shop to measure you.

Braxton Hicks' contractions Painless *contractions* which happen all through *pregnancy.* If they are very strong, the woman may think she is going into *labour* when she is not. This is called false labour.

breast (BREST) A woman or *adolescent* girl has two breasts on her *chest*. A breast is made up of fat and a milk-producing (mammary) *gland*, an *areola* and a *nipple*. A mother's breasts can produce milk for her baby. Breasts are also sensitive to touch and stroking or *kissing* them may increase *sexual* pleasure. Breasts start to develop

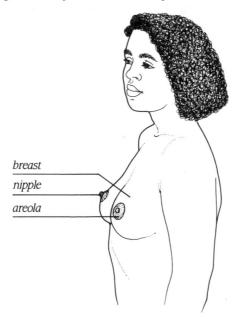

breast

nipple

areola

during *puberty*, usually when the girl is about 11 (although it could be as early as nine or as late as 17). The breasts usually reach their full size by the time the girl is about 17. As the breasts develop, they may hurt a bit and one may grow faster than the other. Many girls and women worry about their breasts being the 'wrong' shape or size but size and shape make no difference to how attractive or sensitive they are, nor to *breastfeeding*. If you are a boy and you think you are starting to develop breasts during puberty, don't worry – the *hormones* causing these changes will settle down and the 'breasts' will disappear within 18 months.

breast milk See *breastfeeding*.

breast self-examination (BSE) Checking your *breasts* for unusual lumps or changes which could be a sign of breast cancer.

For a leaflet on how to examine your breasts, contact the Imperial Cancer Research Fund. Their address is on page 119.

breastfeeding When a mother feeds her baby from her *breasts* rather than from a bottle. When a baby is born, milk is the only 'food' it needs for the first few months. Breast milk is easy for the baby to digest and can help the baby fight off infections. A mother's breasts start to produce milk for her baby three to four days after the *birth* (see *colostrum*). Some women have problems breastfeeding and decide to bottle feed. Other women choose to bottle feed from the start and, as no baby is sucking the milk from their breasts, their own milk dries up.

breech birth The birth of a baby which is born *bottom* first. (Most babies are born head first.) Some breech babies are born by *caesarian section*.

buggery Some people use this word instead of *anal intercourse*.

bum You may find that some people don't like this word. It means *bottom*.

bust The *chest* of a woman or a girl who has reached *puberty*. See *breast*.

buttocks (BUT-erx) The two fleshy cheeks that make up your *bottom*.

C

caesarian section (see-ZAIR-ree-an) The *delivery* of a baby by cutting through a *pregnant* woman's *abdomen* into the *uterus* and lifting the baby out. This is done if the baby cannot be born by being pushed down through the woman's *vagina* (see *labour*). It may be that the woman's *pelvis* is too small, or that the baby needs to be born quickly. In a caesarian birth, the mother is given an *epidural block* or anaesthetic so that she doesn't feel any pain.

candida albicans (KAN-di-da AL-bi-kanz) A yeast which can cause an infection called *thrush*.

cap Some people use this word instead of *diaphragm*.

C

to **caress** (ka-RESS) To touch or stroke affectionately.

celibate (SEL-i-bert) Not having a *sexual relationship*.

cell (SEL) The human body is made up of many millions of tiny units called cells. Each cell is too small to be seen without a microscope. Cells are grouped together into tissues. Groups of tissues form *organs* (such as the *uterus*) and groups of organs form systems (for example, the uterus is part of a woman's *reproductive system*).

cell division The way in which *cells* grow and multiply. If a man's *sperm fertilises* a woman's *ovum* to form a new cell (called a *zygote*), this new cell then divides and divides to form a new human being. So it is by cell division that the fertilised ovum develops into a baby.

cervical cancer (ser-VY-kul or SER-vi-kul) Cancer of the *cervix*.

cervical mucus (ser-VY-kul or SER-vi-kul MEW-kus) A thick, sticky substance in the *cervix*. This mucus gets thinner around the time of *ovulation* so that if *sexual intercourse* takes place, it is easier for the *sperm* to swim through the cervix and *fertilise* the *ovum*. See *natural methods*.

cervical smear test (ser-VY-kul or SER-vi-kul) A test for women aged between 20 and 64 to check for any changes in the *cervix* which could later lead to *cervical cancer*. A doctor can look at the cervix by sliding a plastic or metal instrument called a *speculum* into the woman's *vagina*. A small scraping or smear is taken from the surface of the cervix and tested in a laboratory for unusual *cells*. A smear test is usually painless.

cervix (SER-vix) Part of the *female reproductive system* (see the drawing on page 115). Also called the neck of the womb. The cervix is the strong ring of muscles at the bottom end of the *uterus*. It is closed during *pregnancy* to contain the *fetus* but opens during *labour* so that the baby can leave the uterus and be pushed out through the *vagina*.

change of life Some people use this to mean the *menopause*.

chaste See *chastity*.

chastity (CHASS-ti-ti) When someone has no *sexual contact* with anyone outside *marriage*. Someone like this can be described as chaste.

chest The part of the body which is enclosed by the ribs and breast bone. Some women talk about their chest when they mean their *breasts*.

child abuse See *sexual abuse*.

childbirth Another word for *birth*. See *labour*.

chlamydia (kla-MI-dee-a) A *sexually transmitted infection*. See the table on pages 93 to 96 and *sexually transmitted infection*.

chromosome (KRO-mo-zome) A tiny thread-like structure made up of *genes* which is found in the nucleus of each *cell*. Like all human cells, a *fertilised ovum* contains 46 chromosomes. Two of these are the *sex* chromosomes. The one from the mother is always the same and is called the X chromosome. The one from the father may be an X or a Y chromosome. If the ovum is fertilised by a *sperm* containing an X chromosome, the baby will be a girl (XX). If the ovum is fertilised by a sperm containing a Y chromosome, the baby will be a boy (XY). See the drawing on page 29.

to **circumcise** (SER-kum-size) To remove the *foreskin* from a man's or boy's *penis*. See *circumcision*.

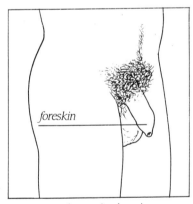
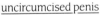
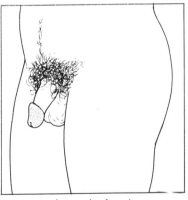

uncircumcised penis   circumcised penis

circumcision (ser-kum-SI-shun) A minor operation to remove the *foreskin* from a man's or boy's *penis*. This is done for religious or medical reasons. Being circumcised makes no difference to *sexual* enjoyment.

the **clap** This word may shock or offend some people. It means *gonorrhoea*.

C

climax (KLY-max) Some people use this word instead of *orgasm*.

clitoris (KLI-tor-iss) The most sensitive part of the *female genitals*. The clitoris is where the inner *labia* meet at the front of the *vulva* (see the drawing on page 115). Only the tip of the clitoris is visible, and it may be covered by a 'hood' or fold of skin. It feels like a small bump about the size of a pea. The clitoris is full of nerve endings and when it is *stimulated* it becomes stiff like an *erect penis* does and pokes out of its hood. Stimulating the clitoris helps many women to have an *orgasm*.

cock This word may shock or offend some people. It means *penis*.

coil Some people use this word instead of *IUD*.

coitus (KOY-tus or KO-ee-tus) This word means *sexual intercourse*.

coitus interruptus See *natural methods*.

colostrum (ko-LOSS-trum) A substance produced by a woman's *breasts* during *pregnancy* and for the first few days after the baby's *birth* before the mother's milk comes into her breasts. It is high in protein and contains *antibodies* which help the baby fight off infections. See *breastfeeding*.

colposcopy (kol-POSS-ko-pi) A medical examination of a woman's *cervix* and the inside of her *vagina* by a lighted magnifying instrument called a colposcope. The examination helps a doctor to look for abnormal (not normal) *cells* around the woman's cervix.

combined pill A method of *contraception* which works by stopping *ovulation* in the woman who takes it. Also called the pill. The combined pill contains two *hormones*, oestrogen and *progestogen*. It is very good at preventing *pregnancy* if the woman follows the instructions on the packet telling her when and how to take it. It also makes her *menstrual periods* very regular and they may be lighter too. Some women who take the

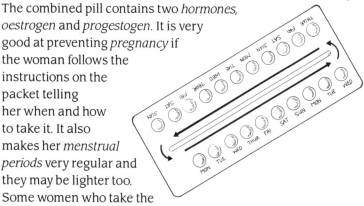

The combined pill

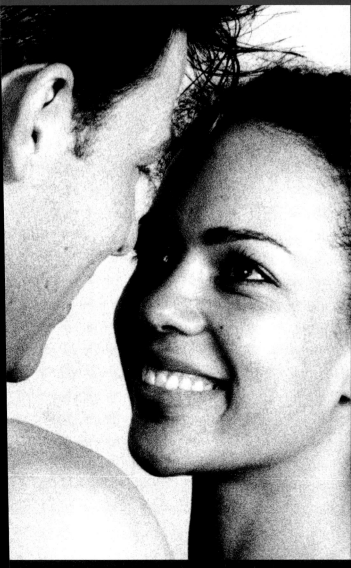

Helping you choose the method of
contraception that is best for you

The combined pill

The combined pill is usually just called the pill. It contains two hormones – oestrogen and progestogen.

These are similar to the natural hormones women produce in their ovaries.

There are a variety of types of combined pill.

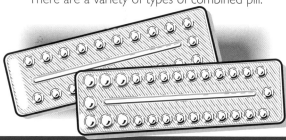

Questions & Answers

How effective is the pill? 3

How does the pill work? 4

Where can I get the pill? 4

Can anyone use the pill? 4

What are the advantages of the pill? 5

What are the disadvantages of the pill? 5

What are the risks of taking the pill? 5

Are all combined pills the same? 7

How do I use EveryDay pills? 8

What if I want to change to a different pill? 8

How to take your 21 day pills and phasic pills 9

Am I protected during the seven day break? 10

What makes the pill less effective? 10

What if I miss a pill and there are less than seven pills left in the pack? 11

pill find that it gives them headaches or sore *breasts*, or makes them feel sick or put on weight. A few have more serious problems such as high blood pressure. For this reason you can only get the pill from a doctor or *family planning clinic* and you need to have regular check-ups. See *contraception*.

to **come** Some people use this word to mean to have an *orgasm* or to *ejaculate*. If a woman 'comes', it means she has an orgasm. If a man 'comes', it means he ejaculates and has an orgasm.

to **come out** To accept that you are *homosexual* or *lesbian*. You may want to let other people know too.

to **conceive** (kon-SEEV) If a woman conceives, it means that one of her *ova* is *fertilised* by a *sperm* from a *male*. This is how a baby starts. See *fertilisation*.

conception (kon-SEP-shun) Some people use this word instead of *fertilisation*.

condom (KON-dom) A condom is a thin rubber sheath which unrolls to fit over a man's *erect penis*. It can be used during *sexual intercourse* between a man and a woman a) to help prevent the woman from becoming *pregnant* (see *contraception*) and b) to lower the risk of *sexually transmitted infection* (see *safer sex*). It can also be used during sexual intercourse between two men to limit the spread of sexually transmitted infections (see *safer sex*). To be effective, a condom must be put on before the penis touches the

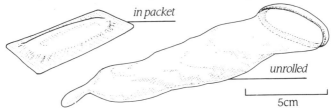

in packet

unrolled

5cm

vaginal or anal area of the other person and it must be kept on the penis until it is fully out of the *vagina* or *anus*. A condom can only be used once. After it has been used, it should be wrapped in a tissue and put in a bin or flushed down the toilet (the tissue stops it floating). With a little practice, condoms are easy to use. They can be bought in many places including chemists and they are free from *family planning clinics*. See *contraception*.

contraception (kon-tra-SEP-shun) Preventing *pregnancy*. Contraception is for men and women who are having *sexual*

C

intercourse and do not want to have a baby. There are nine methods of contraception. They are: 1) *combined pill* 2) *progestogen-only pill* (or 'mini-pill') 3) *injectable contraceptives* 4) *IUD (intra-uterine device)* 5) *diaphragm* (or Dutch cap) plus *spermicide* 6) *contraceptive sponge* 7) *condom* 8) *natural methods* (including the sympto-thermal method) and 9) *sterilisation* of the man or the woman. A tenth method, the *morning-after pill*, is for emergency use only.

The table below shows you how good some of the different methods of contraception are at preventing pregnancy (how reliable they are). All of them have to be used carefully. The first column shows how many women out of a hundred (%) will get pregnant even if they have used that method of contraception <u>very carefully</u> for a year. The second column shows how many women out of a hundred will get pregnant using that method if they are <u>not so careful</u>.

Method	Used very carefully	Used not so carefully
Combined pill	less than 1%	less than 2%
Progestogen-only pill	1%	4%
Diaphragm plus spermicide	2%	15%
Condom	2%	15%
Contraceptive sponge	9%	25%
Sympto-thermal method	2%	20%

Between 1% and 3% of women using an IUD as a method of contraception get pregnant. 1% of women who are given injectable contraceptives as a method of contraception get pregnant. Hardly anyone who has been sterilised gets pregnant.

The condom and diaphragm may also provide protection against *sexually transmitted infections*.

If you have a *relationship* with someone of the opposite *sex* you will not need contraception if you have decided not to have sexual intercourse with them. You may have decided that you do not feel ready for a *sexual relationship* or you may belong to a religious or cultural group that believes that both sex outside *marriage* and contraception are wrong. If you <u>do</u> want to have sexual intercourse but don't want to have a baby, you need to be sure that you won't get 'carried away' and have *unprotected sexual intercourse* by mistake. If you are old enough to have sexual intercourse, you are old enough to talk about contraception with your *partner*, to protect yourselves if necessary from an unwanted pregnancy and to visit your local *family planning clinic* or doctor for help and advice. The law says that if a girl under the age of 16 (below the *age of consent*) asks her doctor for contraception, the doctor should strongly advise the girl to tell her parent(s) or carer(s). But the doctor cannot tell the girl's parent(s) or carer(s) unless the girl agrees to this. The doctor can, however, decide not to treat the girl. For more information about the different methods of contraception, look them up in this dictionary eg 'c' for 'combined pill', 's' for 'sterilisation'. There is also a list of organisations which you can contact for advice on contraception on pages 119 and 120.

contraceptive (kon-tra-SEP-tiv) Something which is used to prevent *pregnancy*. See *contraception*.

contraceptive sponge (kon-tra-SEP-tiv) A method of *contraception* for women. It is a soft, circular sponge containing *spermicide*. The dimple in the sponge fits over the woman's *cervix*. It works as a barrier, stopping *sperm* from getting into the *uterus* and *fertilising* an *ovum*. The spermicide in the sponge also kills sperm in the woman's *vagina*. Before having *sexual intercourse*, the woman wets the sponge with water and puts it into her vagina. The sponge

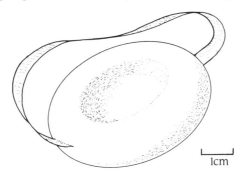

1cm

expands once it is inside her. After intercourse, she leaves the sponge in for at least six hours. To take the sponge out, she gently pulls on the loop which is attached to the sponge. You can buy a contraceptive sponge from a chemist without a doctor's prescription. However, it is not the most reliable method of contraception. It can only be used once and must then be thrown away. See *contraception*.

contraction (kon-TRAK-shun) Tightening of the muscles in the upper part of the *uterus*. Contractions can be a sign for a *pregnant* woman that she is in *labour* (although see *Braxton Hicks' contractions*).

C

In labour, the contractions slowly pull the *cervix* open so that the baby can pass out of the uterus and down into the *vagina*. By the time the cervix is fully open (*dilated*), the contractions may be very strong and they may come every two minutes or so. After the baby is born, another contraction is needed before the *placenta* can be gently pulled out (see *afterbirth*).

to **copulate** Another word which means to have *sexual intercourse*.

crabs You may find that some people don't like this word. It means *pubic lice*.

crotch The area between your legs where the top half of your body stops and your legs start. Also pronounced and spelt 'crutch'. Your crotch includes your *genitals*.

crush Strong feelings of attraction or *desire* for someone. You may have a crush on someone of the same *sex* or the opposite sex. It may be an older girl or boy at school or a teacher. It may be a famous person like a pop star or film star. These feelings can be wonderful but they can also be scary if they are very strong. Crushes are very common in *adolescence* and they are usually a harmless way of exploring new and exciting feelings about other people. As you get older, these kinds of feelings are often replaced by more permanent feelings of *love* and desire.

cum This word may shock or offend some people. It means *semen*.

cunnilingus (kun-i-LIN-gus) See *oral sex*.

cunt This word may shock or offend some people. It means *vulva*.

the **curse** Some people use this word instead of *menstruation* or *menstrual period*.

cystitis (siss-TY-tiss) Inflammation of the *bladder*. Cystitis is more common in women than in men. It can be caused by bacteria which normally live in the *rectum* and around the *anus*. The bacteria can be pushed into the *urethra* and up into the bladder by *sexual intercourse* (see *sexually transmitted infection*), inserting a *tampon*, wiping your *bottom* from back to front, or even just by wearing tight trousers. It can also be caused by an allergic reaction to soap, talc, *vaginal* deodorants etc, friction during sexual intercourse, a sensitive bladder or anxiety and depression. If you have cystitis, you get a burning pain when you pass *urine*, and may have a fever, an ache in your back or lower *abdomen*, and cloudy urine or blood in your urine. Drinking a lot of water, milk, weak orange squash or weak tea can help to flush out the bacteria. If this does not work after a day or two, or if you have blood in your urine, you should see your doctor. The Health Education Authority produces a leaflet on cystitis (their address is on page 119).

D

D & C Stands for dilation and curettage. A simple operation to clean out the *uterus*. The *cervix* is gently opened and the *endometrium* is scraped or sucked away. Women sometimes have a D & C after a *miscarriage*. It is also a method of *abortion*.

deep kissing See *kissing*.

delivery Another word for the *birth* of a baby.

deoxyribonucleic acid See *DNA*.

depo-provera (dep-o-pro-VAIR-a) See *injectable contraceptives*.

desire (di-ZYRE) Desire is a feeling of wanting something. You can have strong feelings of physical desire for someone you are sexually attracted to. These feelings may be strong enough to make you want to have *sexual intercourse* with them.

diaphragm (DY-a-fram) A method of *contraception* for women. Also called the cap or Dutch cap. A diaphragm is a thin rubber dome with a bendy rim. It covers the *cervix* and works as a barrier, stopping *sperm* from getting into the *uterus* and *fertilising* an *ovum*. The woman puts the diaphragm in her *vagina* before having *sexual intercourse*. When it is in the right place, neither the man nor the woman can feel it. To prevent *pregnancy*, the woman also smears it with *spermicide* before putting it in. After intercourse, she leaves it in for at least six hours. She can then take it out, wash it carefully, dry it, and put it away until she needs to use it again. If you choose this method of contraception, you will need to go to a doctor or *family planning clinic* so that you can be fitted with a diaphragm which is exactly the right size for your cervix. You will also have a

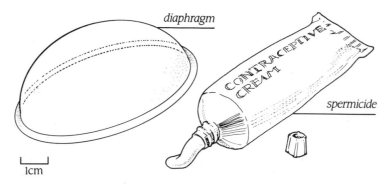

diaphragm

spermicide

1cm

chance to practise putting it in properly and taking it out again. See *contraception*.

dick This word may shock or offend some people. It means *penis*.

dilate (dy-LATE) See *dilation*.

dilation (dy-LAY-shun) The stretching and opening out of a woman's *cervix* during the first stage of *labour*. The cervix has to dilate before the baby can come out of the woman's *uterus*, be pushed down the *vagina* and be born. In a woman who is not pregnant, the cervix is usually about 2mm (⅛in) wide. During labour it stretches to about 10cm (4in) wide.

discharge (DISS-charge) Fluid which comes out of a part of your body. Girls who have reached *puberty* and women usually have some vaginal discharge or wetness (see *vaginal fluid*). Two fluids which come out of a boy's or man's *penis* are *urine* and *semen*. If the discharge from your *vagina* or penis is a strange colour, smells unpleasant, makes you itch or gives you a rash, you could have an infection and you should see your doctor.

divorce (di-VORSS) The legal ending of a *marriage*. Marriages end for many reasons. It may be that one *partner* has found someone else who they think will make them happier. It may be that one partner is violent or very difficult to live with. Or it may just be that the marriage has broken down and the couple no longer want to live together. Most couples separate and live apart for a while before they get divorced. They have to apply to the court for a divorce. Once they are divorced, they are free to marry someone else if they wish. If your parents are thinking about getting divorced, you may be finding your home life quite difficult. There may be arguments and unhappiness between them. You may think that you are to blame. You are not. Your parents' *relationship* has gone wrong, not their love for you. If they do split up you might feel angry, sad or even relieved. If your parents have already separated or divorced, your life could be quite complicated because your parents might be in different places. You may live with one parent and see the other one at weekends or at holiday times. If you find this difficult and it makes you unhappy, try to talk to someone about how you feel. If you can't talk to your parents, try to discuss it with a friend, a teacher who knows you well, or a relative or family friend. Or you could contact one of the organisations which offer counselling for young people. Their addresses are on pages 119 and 120.

DNA Stands for deoxyribonucleic acid. A chemical which is contained in all of our *cells* and is the basic component of the *genes* in our *chromosomes*. To make more cells, a cell divides into two new cells. When a cell divides, the DNA it contains splits into two identical halves, which enter the two new cells. Half the DNA goes into one new cell and the other half goes into the other new cell.

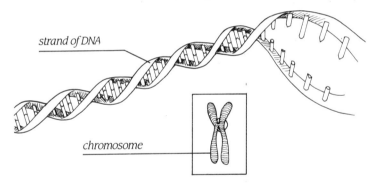

strand of DNA

chromosome

The two new cells therefore contain identical DNA. A cell can reproduce itself exactly in this way many times, with every new cell carrying the same *genetic* information. In a *fertilised ovum*, genes from both parents combine to make a DNA which only that baby will have. This is why everyone is different (but see *identical twins*).

durex (DEW-rex) This is a make of *condom*. Some people use this word instead of condom.

Dutch cap Some people use this to mean *diaphragm*.

dysmenorrhoea (diss-men-er-REE-a) Unusually painful *menstruation*.

E

ectopic pregnancy (ek-TOP-ik) When a *fertilised ovum* starts to grow in a woman's *fallopian tube* instead of in her *uterus*. It causes pain and bleeding in early *pregnancy* and is dangerous. The ovum cannot develop properly and has to be removed in a hospital operation.

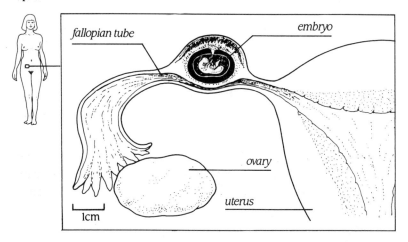

fallopian tube

embryo

ovary

uterus

1cm

egg cell Another term for *ovum*.

ejaculate (i-JAK-u-late) When *semen* spurts out of a man's or boy's *penis* during an *orgasm*. You can only ejaculate when you have reached *puberty* and your *testes* have started to produce *sperm*. As soon as you start to ejaculate, the *bladder* automatically closes so that you cannot pass *urine* and ejaculate at the same time.

ejaculation (i-jak-u-LAY-shun) See *ejaculate*.

embryo (EM-bri-o) An unborn baby during the early stages of *pregnancy* (see the drawing on page 72). After the first eight to 12 weeks of pregnancy, the developing baby is called a *fetus*.

emotion (i-MO-shun) A feeling. Some common emotions are *love*, happiness, anger, sadness, jealousy and hatred. You can experience several different emotions over a short time or even all at once. Swings of emotion are very common during *adolescence*. You might feel up one minute and down the next (see *moods*). This will probably settle down as your *hormones* settle down.

emotional (i-MO-shun-ul) This word describes anything to do with *emotions*. Different things make different people feel emotional. Some people are more emotional than others. Emotional people tend to show their feelings, for example, by crying when they feel sad.

endocrine gland (EN-do-krin) A part of the body which produces natural chemicals called *hormones*. The main endocrine gland is the *pituitary gland*.

endometrium (en-do-MEE-tri-um) The lining of the *uterus*. Each month, as part of the *menstrual cycle*, the endometrium slowly thickens until it is about 5mm (¼in) thick. It also becomes soft and spongy. If a woman becomes *pregnant*, the *fertilised ovum* attaches itself to this lining and starts to develop into a baby. If the *ovum* is not fertilised it passes out of the body along with the lining and some blood (see *menstruation*). Some methods of *contraception* work by making it difficult for a fertilised ovum to attach itself to the endometrium.

epididymis (ep-i-DI-di-miss) Part of the *male reproductive system* (see the drawing on page 114). Two thin coiled tubes, one lying over the back of each *testis*, which store the *sperm* that have been made in the *testes*.

epidural block (ep-i-DUR-al) An injection of local anaesthetic which can be given to a woman during *labour* to make *contractions* hurt less. The woman stays fully awake and alert but because she can no longer feel her *uterus* contracting, the *midwife* may have to tell her when to push in the second stage of labour. This means that sometimes the baby takes longer to be born.

episiotomy (ep-ee-zi-OT-o-mi) A cut which a *midwife* or doctor makes in a woman's *perineum* if her *vaginal opening* will not stretch enough to let the baby's head through at the end of the second stage of *labour*. A local anaesthetic is given before the skin is cut. After the *birth* the cut is stitched up again.

erect (i-REKT) Erect means upright. When a man is *sexually aroused*, blood flows into his *penis* and it becomes hard and stiff. This makes it erect and it goes up at an angle (see *erection* and the drawing on page 114). A boy's penis can also go stiff and hard but when it is erect it does not stick up as much as a man's does. When a woman is sexually aroused, her *clitoris* becomes erect. *Nipples* respond to cold, touch and *sexual arousal* by becoming erect.

erection (i-REK-shun) When a boy's or man's *penis* becomes upright or *erect* (see the drawing on page 114). Boys usually start to get erections more often once they have reached *puberty.* You may get an erection if you are *sexually aroused.* But erections can happen at other times too. You may find that sometimes your penis is slightly erect when you wake up in the morning. This is often because your *bladder* is full and is putting pressure on your penis. When you pass *urine*, the erection soon goes. Even something like the vibrations of a bus or train can give you an erection. This kind of unexpected and unwanted erection can be a bit embarrassing. If this happens to you, think hard about something very boring and the erection should go away.

   When·a man wants to have *penetrative sexual intercourse*, his penis must become erect. After *ejaculation*, he loses his erection and is unlikely to have another one straightaway.

erogenous zones (i-ROJ-er-nus) The areas of your body which make you feel *sexually aroused* when they are touched, stroked or kissed. These include the lips, *breasts, genitals* and *buttocks.* No two people are exactly alike, however, and you may find that other parts of your body make you feel *sexy* when touched.

erotic (i-ROT-ik) Something which makes you feel *sexually aroused* or gives you *sexual* pleasure.

F

facial hair See *hair.*

faeces (FEE-seez) Semi-solid waste matter from your body which comes out through your *anus* when you go to the toilet.

faithful This word means staying loyal to someone or something. In a *sexual relationship*, it means not having *sexual contact* with anyone other than your *partner.*

fallopian tube (fa-LO-pee-an) Part of the *female reproductive system.* There are two fallopian tubes (see the drawing on page 115).

They are muscular tubes, one on each side of the *uterus*. Every month as part of the *menstrual cycle*, an *ovum* is released by one *ovary* into the fallopian tube nearest to it (see *ovulation*). If a woman has *sexual intercourse* with a man around this time, the ovum may be fertilised by a *sperm* in the fallopian tube. See *fertilisation* and *ectopic pregnancy*.

family planning   Some people use this to mean *contraception*.

family planning clinic   A centre where you can get free *contraceptive* advice and supplies. Anyone can go to a family planning clinic – you don't have to be married. There is a list on pages 119 and 120 of organisations which have information about family planning clinics.

fanny   This word may shock or offend some people. It means *vulva*.

to **fantasise** (FAN-ter-size)   To have a *fantasy*.

fantasy (FAN-ter-si)   A fantasy is something you imagine or create in your mind. A *sexual* fantasy is something you imagine which makes you feel *sexually aroused*. Some people enjoy fantasising while they *masturbate*. Sexual fantasies may be about someone you know or they may be about someone you don't know or someone famous. Most fantasies are harmless. They are a way of letting you explore in your mind things which you would probably not do in real life. But if your fantasies start to take over your life and you are no longer sure what is real and what is not, you need help. You can contact one of the counselling organisations on pages 119 and 120 or see your doctor.

fellatio (fer-LAY-shi-o)   See *oral sex*.

female (FEE-male)   A girl or woman. This word is also used to describe something which is a feature of girls or women (as in 'female *genitals*').

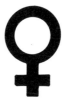

This is the sign for female.

female reproductive system   See *reproductive system*.

female sex hormones   See *sex hormones*.

feminist (FEM-in-ist)   Someone or something supporting equal rights between the sexes.

B

F

fertile (FUR-tile) To be physically able to *conceive* or start a baby. A woman is only fertile once her *reproductive organs* have *matured* and while her *ovaries* can release *ova*. So her fertile years are between *puberty* and the *menopause*. A man is only fertile once his *reproductive organs* have matured and while his *testes* can produce sperm. So his fertile years are from *puberty* until well into old age. But not all men and women are fertile (see *infertile*). Girls who have reached puberty and women are more fertile around the time of *ovulation*.

fertilisation (fur-ti-ly-ZAY-shun) The moment when a *sperm fertilises* an *ovum* and a baby starts. When a man and a woman have *sexual intercourse*, the man puts his *erect penis* into the woman's *vagina*. When he *ejaculates*, a small amount of *semen* containing up

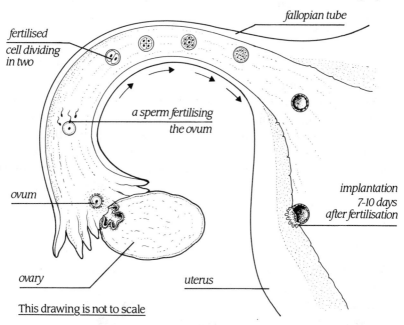

fallopian tube

fertilised cell dividing in two

a sperm fertilising the ovum

ovum

ovary

uterus

implantation 7-10 days after fertilisation

This drawing is not to scale

to 400 million tiny sperm shoots out of the end of his penis and into the woman's vagina. The sperm then swim through the woman's *cervix* into her *uterus*. Some get as far as the woman's *fallopian tubes* where they may meet a *mature ovum* on its way to the uterus (see *ovulation*). Fertilisation takes place if one sperm manages to get through (or penetrate) the outer layer of the ovum and join with the ovum to form a new *cell* called a *zygote*. This new cell will eventually develop into a baby. The woman does not produce any more *ova* while she is *pregnant*, so fertilisation cannot happen again until after she has had the baby. Some methods of *contraception* work by stopping fertilisation from taking place.

fertilise See *fertilisation*.

fertility See *fertile*.

fetus (FEE-tus) An unborn baby which has been developing in a woman's *uterus* for at least eight to 12 weeks. Before this it is called an *embryo*.

fimbria (FIM-bri-a) The fringe-like ends of the *fallopian tubes* (see the drawing on page 115). When *ovulation* takes place and an *ovum* is released, the fimbria sweep the ovum into the fallopian tube.

first stage of labour See *labour*.

flasher A man who shows his *genitals* in public. If a man 'flashes' you in a public place, just ignore him and walk on until you can find someone you can trust and tell them what happened. Flashers tend to be more of a nuisance than a danger.

follicle (FOL-ik-ul) A tiny ball of *cells* in a girl's or woman's *ovary*. A follicle contains an *ovum* (see the drawing on page 65). Follicles play an important part in a girl's or woman's *menstrual cycle*. About every 28 days, between 10 and 20 follicles start to *mature*, producing the *sex hormone oestrogen* as they do so. At the moment of *ovulation*, one follicle bursts open and releases an ovum. The empty follicle is called a corpus luteum (or yellow body). Once it has released the ovum, it starts to produce a second sex hormone, *progesterone*. Oestrogen and progesterone prepare the *endometrium* to receive and nourish a *fertilised* ovum. If the ovum is not fertilised, the ovum, corpus luteum and endometrium start to break down and *menstruation* takes place.

Follicle Stimulating Hormone (FSH) (FOL-i-kul STI-mew-lay-ting HOR-mone) A *hormone* produced by the *pituitary gland* (see the drawing on page 44). In girls who have reached *puberty* and women, FSH (together with another hormone called *Luteinizing Hormone*) makes between 10 and 20 *follicles* start to *mature* at the beginning of each *menstrual cycle* (see *follicle*). It also controls *ovulation*. In boys who have reached puberty and men, FSH makes the *testes* produce *sperm*.

F

fondle (FON-dul) To touch affectionately, squeeze, stroke or *caress*.

fontanelle (fon-tan-EL) The soft spot on top of a baby's head where the skull bones have not yet fused together. This is normal and the bones join up after a year or so. Fontanelle is also spelt 'fontanel'.

forceps (FOR-seps) A surgical instrument which may be used by a doctor in the second stage of *labour* to gently pull the baby out of the mother's *vagina*. Forceps are shaped like a large pair of tongs.

foreplay (FOR-play) *Kissing*, licking and *caressing* in a *sexually arousing* way. Foreplay can happen before *penetrative sexual intercourse* to arouse both *partners*. It can also be a complete sexual act in itself for people who do not want penetrative sexual intercourse.

foreskin (FOR-skin) The skin which covers the tip of the *penis* of a boy or man who has not been *circumcised* (see the drawing on page 21). When the penis is *erect*, the foreskin rolls back, exposing the sensitive tip or *glans*. Boys who have reached *puberty* and men need to wash under their foreskin regularly (see *smegma*).

to **fornicate** (FOR-ni-kate) This word means to have *sexual intercourse* outside *marriage*. Some people use it to mean sexual intercourse that they disapprove of.

fostering A way of providing family life for children who cannot live with their own birth parents for some reason. This could be because their birth parents are ill or have other problems such as no housing or no work. Fostering is not the same as *adoption*. It is usually for a short time – weeks, months or a few years at the most. If you are fostered, your foster parents will look after you on a day-to-day basis but they will share the caring with your birth parents who may visit you regularly. If you are staying with a foster family, you may find it difficult being away from your own family. But sharing the security, *love* and ups and downs of your foster family can be a very good experience too. For more information about fostering, contact the British Agencies for Adoption and Fostering (BAAF). Their address is on page 119.

French kissing See *kissing*.

French letter Some people use this to mean *condom*.

frigid (FRI-jid) Someone who cannot be *sexually aroused*. This doesn't necessarily mean they don't have *sexual* feelings. They may just be in the wrong situation or with the wrong person when they have *sexual contact*.

frottage See *safer sex*.

FSH Stands for *Follicle Stimulating Hormone*.

to **fuck** This word may shock or offend some people. It means to have *sexual intercourse*.

G

gamete (GA-meet) Another word for a *sperm* or an *ovum*.

gang bang This word may shock or offend some people. A gang bang is when a woman is *raped* by several men one after the other. See *rape*.

gas and air A method of pain relief for women during *labour* and *birth*. The woman breathes in a mixture of oxygen and another gas called nitrous oxide through a mask which she holds over her mouth and nose. This helps some women cope with very strong *contractions*.

gay Some people use this word to mean *homosexual* or *lesbian*.

gender (JEN-der) Your sex – whether you are *male* or *female*.

genes (JEENZ) Genes determine our individual characteristics as people. They are made up of *DNA* and we inherit them from our parents. Genes exist like a string of beads in *chromosomes* which are found in each *cell*. There are about 2,000 genes in each chromosome and 46 chromosomes in each cell. 23 chromosomes are passed on by the mother and the other 23 come from the father. We can't change the genes we are born with so we have the same ones for the whole of our lives. They determine things like our blood group, height, build, and eye and hair colour. They may also affect things like personality and intelligence but the way we are brought up and the way we live have an effect on these things too.

G

genetic (jer-NET-ik) A word to describe something to do with *genes*. Sometimes an abnormal (not normal) gene which causes health or mental problems is passed on. If someone inherits a genetic problem and then has a child, they may in turn pass it on to the child. So if someone with a genetic problem wants to have a baby, a doctor can give them advice on the chances of the baby inheriting the problem. This is called genetic counselling.

genetics (jer-NET-ix) The study of *genes* and how inherited characteristics are passed on by parents to their children.

genital (JEN-i-tul) The genitals are the *sex organs* which are outside the body (see the drawings on pages 114 and 115). *Male* genitals include the *penis* and *scrotum*. *Female* genitals include the *labia*, the *clitoris* and the *vaginal opening*. The *vulva* is another word for the female genitals.

genital herpes (JEN-i-tul HER-peez) A *sexually transmitted infection*. See the table on pages 93 to 96 and *sexually transmitted infection*.

genital warts (JEN-i-tul) A *sexually transmitted infection*. See the table on pages 93 to 96 and *sexually transmitted infection*.

genito-urinary clinic (JEN-i-to-YEW-rin-ri) Some people use this to mean *Special Clinic*.

genito-urinary infection (JEN-i-to-YEW-rin-ri) An infection which affects the *genitals* or the parts of the body through which *urine* passes (the *bladder* and the *urethra*). Many genito-urinary infections are *sexually transmitted*. See *sexually transmitted infection*.

German measles Some people use this to mean *rubella*.

gestation (jess-TAY-shun) The time taken for an unborn baby to develop in its mother's *uterus*. Gestation in humans is about nine months.

to get it up This phrase may shock or offend some people. It means to have an *erection* or to have *sexual intercourse*.

gigolo (JIG-o-lo) A man who is paid by women to go out with them. Some gigolos are also paid to *have sex* with women.

give birth See *labour* and *birth*.

gland A part of the body which produces a substance needed by the body to work properly. For example, sweat glands produce sweat, which the body needs to keep its temperature right.

Sebaceous glands produce *sebum* which helps to keep your hair and skin waterproof and your skin supple. Mammary glands in a mother's *breasts* can produce milk for her baby. In men, the *prostate gland* and Cowpers' glands produce a substance which *stimulates sperm* into making swimming movements. *Endocrine glands* produce special natural chemicals called *hormones.*

glans The tip of the *penis* or *clitoris* (see the drawings on pages 114 and 115). The glans has many nerve endings which make it the most sensitive part of both the *female* and the *male genitals.*

to **go all the way** Some people use this to mean to have *sexual intercourse.*

to **go to bed with someone** Some people use this to mean to have *sexual intercourse* with someone.

gonorrhoea (gon-o-REE-a) A *sexually transmitted infection.* See the table on pages 93 to 96 and *sexually transmitted infection.*

growth spurt Growing a lot over a short period of time. This happens to very young children and again during *puberty,* when the

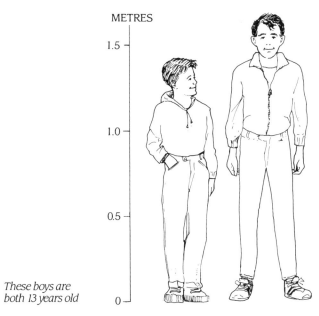

METRES

1.5

1.0

0.5

0

These boys are both 13 years old

pituitary gland sends growth *hormones* around the body. Girls tend to start their growth spurt at around 10 or 11 years but it varies from person to person. The main growth spurt for boys tends to start later, at around 12 or 13 years, but again it varies. By the age of about 14, boys have usually caught up with girls and may go on growing for a year or so after girls have reached their adult height at about 17 years. How tall you are has more to do with the *genes* you have inherited from your parents than how old you are when your growth spurt starts. Not all boys and girls have a spurt of growth; some grow taller gradually.

GU   Stands for *genito-urinary.*

gynaecologist (gy-na-KOL-o-jist)   A doctor who specialises in women's health problems.

H

haemorrhoids (HEM-er-roydz)   Swollen veins near or inside the *anus.* Also called 'piles'. You can get haemorrhoids if you are constipated and have to strain when you go to the toilet. A woman can also get them when she is *pregnant* and after the *birth* of her baby. Haemorrhoids can be painful and they may bleed. You can buy special creams at the chemist to make them hurt less. Your doctor can give you an injection for haemorrhoids or you can have a hospital operation to remove them.

hair   Hair grows on our heads and our bodies. During *puberty, sex hormones* cause more hair to grow, especially around the *genitals* (see *pubic hair*) and under the arms. Boys also start to grow more hair on their face (facial hair) and sometimes on their chest. They can either shave off the facial hair (see *shaving*) or decide to grow a moustache or beard. Girls sometimes also get a fine covering of facial hair once they reach puberty but they should not shave it off. If a girl's facial hair is very dark, she can use a hair removing cream from the chemist or ask a beauty expert about removing the hair by electrolysis or dying it a lighter colour. Some women remove the hair from their legs and from under their arms using a cream or a razor but there is no need to do this if you don't want to. During puberty, the sebaceous *glands* in your skin start to produce more *sebum.* This can make the hair on your head greasy and you may find that you have to wash it more often.

hand job You may find that some people don't like this expression. It means *masturbation*.

hard on You may find that some people don't like this expression. It means *erection*.

to **have a baby** See *labour* and *birth*.

to **have a period** Some people use this to mean to *menstruate*.

to **have it off** You may find that some people don't like this expression. To have it off with someone means to have *sexual intercourse* with them.

to **have sex** Some people use this to mean to have *sexual intercourse*.

heavy petting *Kissing*, touching and cuddling in a *sexual* way. Two people who are heavy petting may explore each other's mouths with their tongues and touch each other's *breasts* and/or *genitals*. They may become *sexually aroused* but probably do not go on to have *sexual intercourse*. Heavy petting can be very exciting and it can give you a lot of pleasure. But it can also be scary if you are not sure whether you want to do it. If your partner wants you to take part in some heavy petting and you don't want to, say so. It's your body.

height See *growth spurt*.

hepatitis B (hep-a-TY-tiss BEE) A form of hepatitis infection which is mainly *sexually transmitted*. See the table on pages 93 to 96 and *sexually transmitted infection*.

heredity (hi-RED-i-ti) Passing on an inherited characteristic from one generation to another. See *DNA* and *genes*.

herpes (HER-peez) An infection caused by the herpes simplex virus (HSV). There are two types of HSV. HSV1 causes cold sores on the lips, face and mouth. HSV2 causes sores in the *genital* area. For this reason it is also called *genital herpes*. See the table on pages 93 to 96 and *sexually transmitted infection*.

heterosexist (het-er-o-SEX-ist) Someone who believes or something that encourages the belief that everyone is *heterosexual*.

heterosexual (het-er-o-SEX-you-ul) A word used to describe someone who has *sexual* feelings towards someone of the opposite *sex*.

H

HIV Stands for human immunodeficiency virus. HIV is the virus which can cause *AIDS*. It is found in *body fluids* such as blood, *semen, vaginal fluid* and *breast milk*. (It is also found in saliva, but not in enough quantity to infect you. You would have to swallow

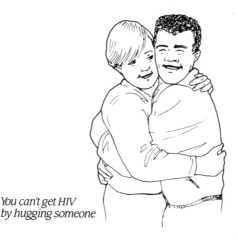

You can't get HIV by hugging someone

pints of saliva to become infected in this way.) HIV can be passed on if body fluids from an infected person get into another person's body. There are three main ways in which this can happen:

1 Having *vaginal* or *anal intercourse* with an infected person without using a *condom*
2 Sharing needles and other equipment for injecting drugs with an infected person
3 A mother with HIV can pass the virus on to her baby in *pregnancy,* at *birth* or through her breast milk.

Some people have been infected with the virus through blood transfusions and other blood products but this is now very unlikely in the UK because all blood and blood products are checked for the virus before they are used. In some countries where you can't easily get sterilised needles and blood products this is still a problem.

You can't tell just by looking at someone whether or not they have HIV. They may not even know themselves. So before you have *sexual contact* with someone, you need to think about how you can lower the risk of being infected. See *safer sex*.

In theory, there is a risk in *oral sex, French kissing* or *deep kissing* with someone who is HIV-infected if you have a cut or sore in your mouth. This is because the virus could pass directly into your bloodstream through the cut or sore. The virus might also pass into your bloodstream if you have acupuncture, a tattoo or your ears pierced and there is infected blood on the needle. In practice, however, the risk of being infected in these ways is very low.

There is no risk in *kissing*, stroking, hugging or having close physical contact with someone who has HIV. And HIV cannot be passed on from cups, cutlery, glasses, food, clothes, towels, toilet seats, door knobs, sneezing, coughing, swimming pools, tears, sweat, mosquitoes or other insects.

If you are worried about HIV or AIDS, you can telephone the National AIDS Helpline. Their telephone number is on page 120.

HIV antibody test (AN-ti-bo-di) A blood test which looks for *antibodies* to *HIV*. It tells you whether you have been infected with HIV. It does not tell you if you have *AIDS* or if you will go on to develop AIDS. If antibodies to HIV are found in your blood, you are 'HIV antibody positive' (HIV AB+) or 'HIV positive'. If you think you might be HIV-infected and should have a test, telephone the National AIDS Helpline. They can tell you the advantages and disadvantages of having a test and the best place to go for a test if you decide to have one. Their telephone number is on page 120.

HIV positive See *HIV antibody test*.

holding back Some people use this to mean coitus interruptus. See *natural methods*.

homophobia (hom-o-FO-bi-a) Fear of *homosexuals* and homosexuality.

homosexual (ho-mo-SEX-you-ul) Someone who is sexually attracted to someone of the same sex, although not many people use the word to describe women who are sexually attracted to other women (see *lesbian*). The word homosexual is generally used to describe a man who is sexually attracted to another man although most homosexual men prefer to describe themselves as *gay* men. Many people do not approve of two men having close physical contact or a *sexual relationship*, so being a homosexual is not always easy. A man and a woman who are having a *relationship* usually feel free to hold hands in public, go where they want, and be open with their family and friends about the fact that they are a couple. But if two men are having a relationship with each other, it can be more difficult for them to do things like this.

H

During *adolescence*, you may experience strong feelings for another boy. This is quite common and you are not a homosexual just because you have these feelings. Nine out of ten times, these feelings disappear. But as many as one in ten boys or men is homosexual. Even if you think you may be a homosexual, it can still take time to be sure about it. This may be a difficult time for you and support from friends, family and possibly other homosexuals will be important.

If two men are having a sexual relationship, they might decide to have *anal intercourse*. If so, they need to think about ways of protecting themselves from the risk of *HIV* infection and other *sexually transmitted infections*. See *anal intercourse* and *safer sex*.

If you think you might be a homosexual, you can talk to someone about it at one of the organisations listed on pages 119 and 120.

hormone (HOR-mone) A natural chemical made by an *endocrine gland*. Different hormones affect different parts of the body. They

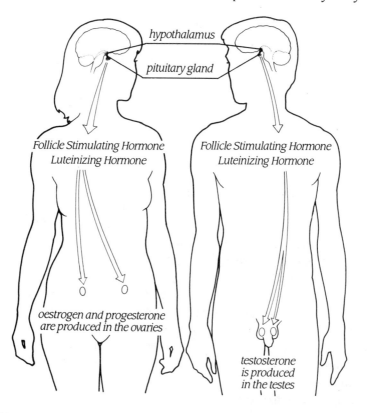

travel around the body in your blood. Hormones control things like your growth and *sexual* development (see *sex hormone*).

hormone replacement therapy (HRT) (HOR-mone ri-PLAYSS-ment THE-ra-pi) Treatment for women who have problems while they are going through the *menopause*. The woman takes the *hormones oestrogen* and/or *progestogen*, usually as tablets or injections.

horny You may find that some people don't like this word. It means *sexually aroused* and wanting to *have sex*.

hot flush A sudden and brief feeling of heat in the face or across the top half of a woman's body. The woman may also sweat heavily. Many women who are going through the *menopause* have hot flushes. They are caused by *hormone* changes. They are not harmful but some women find them a nuisance and may be embarrassed by them.

HRT Stands for *hormone replacement therapy.*

human immunodeficiency virus See *HIV.*

hymen (HY-men) A very thin membrane or layer of skin which covers part of the *vaginal opening* (see the drawing on page 115). Every girl's or woman's hymen is different. Some people have hymens which look complete but which contain enough tiny holes to let *menstrual blood* through when they have their *menstrual period*. Some religious and cultural groups expect a woman to have a complete hymen when she gets married. This is because one way in which a hymen is broken is through having *sexual intercourse.* If her hymen is broken, they say she can't be a *virgin.* But putting a *tampon* in your vagina can also break your hymen. So can riding a bike or a horse or doing a lot of sport, gym or dancing.

hypothalamus (hy-per-THAL-a-muss) A tiny part of your brain which is very close to the *pituitary gland* (see the drawing on page 44). *Puberty* begins when the hypothalamus produces *hormones* (called releasing factors) which trigger the pituitary gland into making hormones of its own.

hysterectomy (hiss-ter-REK-to-mi) When a woman has her *uterus* removed in a hospital operation. She cannot have a baby after she has had a hysterectomy.

I

identical twins See *twins*.

illegitimate (i-li-JIT-er-mut) An illegitimate person is someone whose parents were not married when she or he was born.

immoral (i-MO-rul) This word means something which is against the morals or acceptable behaviour of society. Some people use it to describe *sexual activity* which they disapprove of.

immune system (i-MEWN) The body's system for defending itself against infections and disease. *HIV (human immunodeficiency virus)* destroys the immune system so that a person with HIV is less able to fight off infections.

implantation (im-plarn-TAY-shun) When a *fertilised ovum* attaches itself to the *endometrium* (see the drawing on page 34). This usually happens between seven and ten days after *fertilisation*. Once implantation has taken place, the woman is *pregnant*.

impotence (IM-po-tenss) When a man cannot get or keep an *erection* or *ejaculate*. This sometimes happens when a man is worried or under stress or it may be a physical problem. Impotence is very common and there is usually no need to worry. However, if a man is having regular *sexual intercourse* and finds that he is always impotent, he should see his doctor.

impotent See *impotence*.

in vitro fertilisation (in VEE-tro) See *IVF*.

incest (IN-sest) *Sexual intercourse* between two people who are closely related to each other, for example, a father and daughter, a brother and sister, an uncle and niece or a mother and son. Incest is against the law in the UK. It is also something which people tend not to talk about, perhaps because they are frightened or don't want to get the other person into trouble. If someone close to you in your family is making you do sexual things with them, it is important that you turn to page 86 and read what it says under *sexual abuse*.

induce See induction.

induction (in-DUK-shun) When *labour* is started artificially (or induced). This is sometimes done because there is a risk to the

46

unborn baby or to the mother's health. Perhaps the baby is overdue or the mother has high blood pressure. Labour is started by breaking the *amniotic sac* or by using drugs to start the *contractions*.

infatuation (in-fat-you-AY-shun) When you have an infatuation you are unrealistically crazy about someone. You probably think about them all the time. Your strong feelings may blind you to their faults and to the reality of the situation. You may prefer your image of that person to the real thing! This could make a relationship with them very difficult. If someone is infatuated with you it is better to keep your distance and not take advantage of their strong feelings for you.

infertile (in-FER-tyle) A person who is unable to start a baby. A man who is infertile (or *sterile*) may be producing *sperm* which are not healthy enough to *fertilise* an *ovum*. A woman who is infertile (or sterile) may not be producing an ovum each month (see *ovulation*). Another reason why both men and women can be infertile is that the tubes down which the sperm and *ova* travel (the *vas deferens* in men and the *fallopian tubes* in women) may be blocked or damaged. This means that the sperm cannot reach the ovum and *fertilisation* cannot take place inside the woman's body. Nowadays, this problem can sometimes be overcome by *IVF (in vitro fertilisation)*.

infertility clinic A clinic where men and women who are finding it difficult to start a baby can go for help. See *infertile*.

inherited characteristics Features which are passed on (or inherited) from our parents. See *genes*.

injectable contraceptives A method of *contraception* which is used as a last resort for women who find all other methods impossible to use. There are two injectable contraceptives – depo-provera and noristerat. They are both *progestogens*. They are injected into a *buttock* or an arm muscle by a doctor every two or three months. Women injected with these progestogens can experience serious problems with their *menstrual periods, fertility,* weight and mental health, and may be more likely to get *cervical cancer.* See *contraception*.

inner labia See *labia*.

intercourse See *sexual intercourse*.

internal examination Internal means inside. An internal examination is when a doctor examines a girl's or woman's *reproductive organs*. The doctor sometimes uses a *speculum* so that she or he can see the inside of the *vagina* and the *cervix*. The doctor may also do a bimanual examination. To do this the doctor puts on a clean polythene glove and slides two fingers of one hand into the woman's vagina, putting the other hand on the woman's lower *abdomen*. By pressing and feeling between the two hands, the doctor can check the woman's *uterus* and *ovaries* for any problems. A doctor may also do a bimanual examination to confirm that a woman is *pregnant*.

intimate (IN-ter-mut) This word means very close and personal. Intimate contact with someone can mean *sexual contact*.

intra-uterine device See *IUD*.

the **itch** You may find that some people don't like this word. It means *scabies*.

IUD Stands for intra-uterine device. A method of *contraception* for women. An IUD is a small piece of plastic which sometimes has thin copper wire around part of it. It works by making it difficult for a *fertilised ovum* to attach itself to the *endometrium*. A doctor puts it

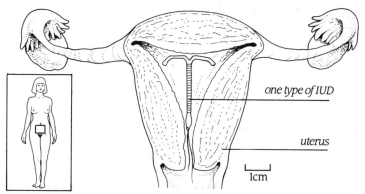

one type of IUD

uterus

1cm

into the *uterus* through the *vagina*. Cotton threads hang down from it and every now and then the woman should feel for the threads inside her vagina to check that the IUD is still in her uterus. The IUD is good at stopping a woman from becoming *pregnant* and it only needs to be changed every three to five years. However, it can cause heavy or painful *menstrual periods* and there is an increased risk of infection of the uterus or *fallopian tubes*. See *contraception*.

IVF Stands for in vitro fertilisation. *Fertilisation* of an *ovum* by a *sperm* outside a woman's body. Fertilisation takes place in a

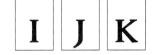
laboratory rather than in the woman's *fallopian tube*. The fertilised ovum is then put back into the woman's *uterus*. If *implantation* takes place, the fertilised ovum develops into a baby in the same way as in a normal *pregnancy*. IVF is a way of helping a couple who are finding it difficult to start a baby. It is a delicate process which does not always work. Some people call a baby started in this way a 'test tube' baby.

J

jealous (JEL-us) Wanting to have someone all to yourself and being afraid of losing their *love* and affection.

to **jerk off** This expression may shock or offend some people. It means to *masturbate*.

johnny Some people use this word instead of *condom*.

K

kissing A way of expressing *love* or affection or greeting someone with a touch of the lips. You and your friends and family may touch,

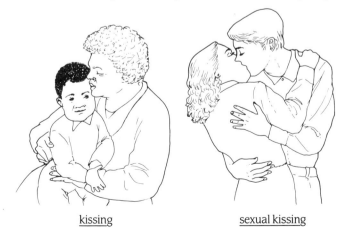

kissing   sexual kissing

hug and kiss each other. But kissing sexually (deep kissing or French kissing) is when two people part their lips and their tongues play inside each other's mouth. It can make both people feel *sexually aroused* and make them want to have *sexual intercourse* together. If two people are having a *sexual relationship,* they can kiss any part of each other's body which gives them both pleasure. This may include their *genitals* (see *oral sex*).

knob You may find that some people don't like this word. It means *penis.*

knockers You may find that some people don't like this word. It means *breasts.*

KY jelly (KAY-WY JEL-i) A lubricating jelly which you can buy from a chemist. See *lubricate.* KY jelly is not a *spermicide* so it can't stop you getting *pregnant.*

L

labia (LAY-bee-a) A Latin word meaning 'lips'. The labia are part of a girl's or woman's *genitals* (see the drawing on page 115). There are two types of labia – the outer labia and the inner labia. The outer labia (labia majora) are the two fatty folds of skin between a girl or woman's legs. *Pubic hair* grows over the outer labia of girls who have reached *puberty* and women. The outer labia are normally closed so that they can protect the more delicate parts underneath them such as the *vagina* and the *clitoris.* The inner labia (labia minora) are thinner than the outer labia and they can be seen when the outer labia are parted. They are sensitive to touch and they swell and darken in colour when a woman is *sexually aroused.*

labour (LAY-ber) The process by which a baby leaves its mother's body to be born. A *pregnant* woman knows her labour is beginning when she has regular *contractions,* a 'show', or when her waters break (see *amniotic fluid*). Labour happens in three stages:

First stage of labour
In the first stage of labour, the *cervix,* which is closed with a plug of mucus during *pregnancy,* opens up. Strong muscular contractions of the *uterus* help

this to happen, but it can still take between two and 12 hours for the cervix to stretch enough to let the baby out (see *dilation*).

Second stage of labour

In the second stage of labour, which ends with the baby's *birth*, the baby passes out of the uterus and down the woman's *vagina* (although see *caesarian section*). The woman has to push hard with each contraction until

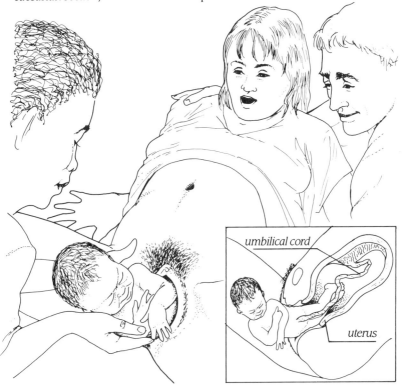

umbilical cord

uterus

the baby's head starts to come out through her *vaginal opening*. She might have to have an *episiotomy* and/or *forceps* at this stage if the baby is not coming out easily. Once the head is born, the rest of the baby's body usually slides out very quickly (although see *breech birth*). As soon as the baby is born and is breathing properly the *umbilical cord* is cut and clamped. Then the mother can hold and cuddle the baby and let it suck at her *breast* if she wants to.

Third stage of labour

The third stage of labour often happens without the mother realising it because she is too busy getting to know her new baby. In this stage, the *placenta* leaves the mother's body (see *afterbirth*). Some mothers are given a special injection to make this stage happen quickly.

L

Labour can be exhausting and painful, although there are lots of ways of making it hurt less (see *epidural block, gas and air* and *pethidine*). For many women (and men), however, the birth of their baby is such a wonderful moment that they forget about all the hard work of giving birth.

Sometimes, labour ends sadly with the baby born dead (a *stillbirth*) or dying. If this happens, the parents can get help and counselling from the Stillbirth and Neonatal Death Association. Their address is on page 120.

laparoscopy (la-pa-ROSS-ko-pi) An examination of a woman's *uterus, fallopian tubes* and *ovaries* using an instrument called a laparoscope. The doctor puts the laparoscope through a small cut about 1cm (³⁄₈in) long close to the woman's *navel*. Laparoscopy can be used in *female sterilisation* and to diagnose problems in a woman's *pelvic* area.

lesbian (LEZ-bee-an) A woman who is sexually attracted to another woman. Some lesbians prefer to describe themselves as *gay*. Many people do not approve of two women having close physical contact or a *sexual relationship*, so being a lesbian is not always easy. A man and a woman who are having a *relationship* usually feel free to hold hands in public, go where they want, and be open with their family and friends about the fact that they are a couple. But if two women are having a relationship with each other, it can be more difficult for them to do things like this.

During *adolescence*, you may experience strong feelings for another girl. This is quite common and you are not a lesbian just because you have these feelings. Nine out of ten times, these feelings disappear. But as many as one in ten girls or women is lesbian. Even if you think you may be a lesbian, it can still take time to be sure about it. This may be a difficult time for you and support from friends, family and possibly other lesbians will be important.

If you think you might be a lesbian, you can talk to someone about it at one of the organisations listed on pages 119 and 120.

LH Stands for *Luteinizing Hormone*.

libido (li-BEE-do) Your sex drive – the intensity of your *sexual* feelings and how *sexually active* you are. Your libido is affected by your *sex hormones*. It is also affected by the situation you are in. For example, being unhappy in a *relationship*, or feeling guilty, shy, frightened or very tired, can lower your libido.

lining of the uterus Some people use this to mean *endometrium*.

lips (inner and outer) See *labia*.

love A powerful feeling of affection, attachment or *sexual desire*. Love is one of the most basic human *emotions* and it has inspired writers and poets for hundreds of years. There are many different kinds of love. There is *platonic* love which you might feel for people in your family, for friends of the same or opposite *sex* or even for a pet. There is religious love. And there is the love you might feel for someone you are sexually attracted to, which can make you want to share your life and everything that you have with that person. People often say that they love something if they like it very much but loving a person is more complicated than this. If you love someone, you may want to do things for them, look after them and protect them, confide in them, listen to them, share things with them, spend time with them, *have sex* with them, marry them, have children with them. You may find that there are times when you have to put their needs first and perhaps give something up for them. Love of this kind can develop very gradually or you might fall in love suddenly and quickly. Don't worry if your experience of loving and being loved isn't the same as everyone else's. We are all different and so we experience love in different ways too.

to lubricate (LOO-bri-kate) To make slippery. When a woman is *sexually aroused*, her *vagina* becomes moist or lubricated. If she is going to have *penetrative sexual intercourse* with a man, this makes it easier for his *penis* to slide into her vagina. Some *condoms* are lubricated for the same reason. A woman can use a lubricating jelly like *KY jelly* if her vagina is rather dry.

Luteinizing Hormone (LH) (LOO-ti-nize-ing HOR-mone) A *hormone* produced by the *pituitary gland* (see the drawing on page 44). Each month during the *menstrual cycle* of a girl who has reached *puberty* or a woman, LH (together with another hormone called *Follicle Stimulating Hormone*) controls *ovulation*. After ovulation, LH also makes the empty *follicle* produce the *female sex hormone progesterone*. In boys who have reached puberty and men, LH makes the *testes* start to produce higher levels of the *male sex hormone testosterone*.

M

macho (MATCH-O) A word to describe a man who is, or likes to think he is, very tough and manly. It comes from the Spanish word 'machismo', which means *male*.

maidenhead (MAY-den-hed) Some people use this to mean *hymen*.

to make love Some people use this to mean to have *sexual intercourse*.

male A boy or man. This word is also used to describe something which is a feature of boys or men (as in 'male genitals').

This is the sign for male.

male chauvinist (SHO-ver-nist) A boy or man who thinks girls or women are inferior and who treats them as such.

male reproductive system See *reproductive system*.

male sex hormones See *sex hormones*.

mammary gland See *breast*.

marriage (MA-rij) When a man and woman become husband and wife. People usually get married in a registry office or in a place of worship. People who live together but who are not married are sometimes called common-law wife and husband. You must be at least 16 to get married. In England, Wales and Northern Ireland, if you want to get married in a registry office before the age of 18 you need the written permission of your parent(s) or guardian(s). In Scotland you don't need this permission. The decision to get married is usually made by the couple themselves. In some cultures, however, the marriage is arranged by the parents of the couple. Many marriages are very happy and successful but not all marriages last for life (see *divorce*).

masochist (MASS-o-kist) Someone who enjoys being hurt. A masochist finds it sexually exciting when their *sexual partner* hurts them. Most people do not enjoy *sex* with pain.

massage See *safer sex*.

mastectomy (mass-TEK-tom-i) A hospital operation to remove a woman's *breast* (or both breasts). This may be done if the woman has breast cancer.

masturbate See *masturbation*.

masturbation (mass-ter-BAY-shun) Causing *sexual* excitement and pleasure by rubbing your own (or your *sexual partner's*) *penis* or *clitoris*. There are different ways of masturbating. Boys and men often hold the *shaft* of their penis in their hand and move their hand rhythmically up and down. Girls and women may use their fingers or hand to rub their clitoris. You can also masturbate your sexual partner by doing this for them. Masturbating can give you good feelings and it can make you sexually excited enough to have an *orgasm*. It can also help you get to know your own body. You should, however, only do it in private as it will offend other people if you do it in public. There are lots of stories about terrible things that happen to people who masturbate – they go mad, go blind, can't have babies, grow hairs on the palms of their hands etc. These stories are <u>not true</u>. Masturbating can't do you any harm and there is no need to feel guilty or scared about it. But some people never feel the need to masturbate. This doesn't mean that they can't enjoy *sex*. Other people don't want to masturbate because their religion or *morals* say that it is wrong.

maternal (mat-ERN-ul) This word is used to describe something which is a feature of a mother (as in 'maternal *love*' for a child).

mature (ma-CHORE) To be physically mature means that your body has done its growing and that you are an adult. To be sexually mature means that the *sexual* parts of your body (your *reproductive organs* and *genitals*) are fully developed and that you are physically capable of starting a baby. But just because your body is sexually mature, it doesn't mean that you have to rush off, have *sex* and start a baby. These things can wait until you're ready. (For many people this means until they are married.) To be *emotionally* mature means that you have developed your own views and feelings about things and that you are capable of using your experience to make your own decisions and judgements. Mature can also simply mean 'older'. It is also used to describe an *ovum* which is ready to be released from an *ovary* (see *ovulation*) or a *sperm* which is ready to leave a man's body when he *ejaculates* and which could *fertilise* an ovum.

maturity See *mature.*

menarche (men-ARK) A girl's first *menstrual period.*

menopause (MEN-o-pawz) When a woman in middle age stops *ovulating* and having *menstrual periods.* A woman can't get *pregnant* after the menopause. The menopause may last for some years. Most women start the menopause when they are about 50 years old, but it can happen any time between the ages of 40 and 55. A woman's menstrual periods may be irregular for a year or two before they actually stop. Women going through the menopause often have *hot flushes*, night sweats and vaginal dryness. They may also find that their *emotions* and personality are affected during the menopause and that they become irritable or depressed. Some women find the menopause hard to cope with because of how it affects their bodies and feelings. Other women are pleased to reach the menopause because it means no more menstrual periods and no more worries about getting pregnant.

menstrual blood See *menstrual flow.*

menstrual cycle (MEN-strew-ul SY-kul) The monthly process in which the *female reproductive organs* get ready for the possibility of *pregnancy.* The main events in the menstrual cycle are *ovulation*, the thickening of the *endometrium* and *menstruation.* The length of a menstrual cycle can be anything from 20 to 36 days but the average cycle is about 28 days long. A woman who starts to menstruate at 13, stops at 50 and has two children, could have more than 400 menstrual cycles in her lifetime! When you start menstruating your menstrual cycles are often not very regular. You may only menstruate three or four times in the first year. A middle-aged woman's menstrual cycle may also become irregular before she starts the *menopause.* Stress, shock, worry or excitement can affect your cycle and may make your *menstrual periods* come late or early or stop them altogether (see *amenorrhoea*). If you have regular menstrual cycles and you want to know when to expect your next menstrual period, you can keep a note of when you start your menstrual period each month.

menstrual flow (MEN-strew-ul) The fluid that comes out of a girl's or woman's *vagina* during her *menstrual period.* It looks like blood but it is actually menstrual blood mixed with *cervical mucus*, *vaginal fluid, cells* and broken down bits of the *endometrium*. Most girls or women lose about four to six tablespoons of menstrual fluid each time they menstruate (see *menstruation*). Most of it comes out during the first three days of the menstrual period. You can soak up the menstrual flow with *sanitary towels*, pads or *tampons*. Menstrual flow can start to smell once it is outside the body so it is important to stay fresh by washing your *genital* area and changing towels or pads regularly. Tampons should be changed regularly too (see *sanitary towel* and *tampon*).

menstrual period (MEN-strew-ul PEER-i-od) The time when a girl or woman is menstruating (see *menstruation*). A menstrual period usually lasts between two and eight days and happens about once a month. If you have had *unprotected sexual intercourse* and your menstrual periods stop, you might be *pregnant* and should see a doctor.

menstruate See *menstruation*.

menstruation (men-strew-AY-shun) The monthly *discharge* of blood from a girl's or woman's *uterus*. Menstruation is absolutely normal and healthy. The blood that comes out of your *vagina* is not a sign that anything is wrong. A girl starts to menstruate when she begins *puberty*. This can be any time between the ages of nine and 18. The average age is probably about 13. To menstruate, a girl needs to weigh about 47.5kg or 7½ stone. To menstruate regularly, she needs to be slightly heavier than this. Menstruation usually happens every month between *puberty* and the *menopause* but not while you are *pregnant* or *breastfeeding*. It happens because *sex hormones* make the *endometrium* grow thicker and get soft and spongy, ready to receive a *fertilised ovum* (see *fertilisation*). If no ovum is fertilised, the thickened endometrium is not needed so it breaks away from the uterus and passes out of the vagina together with a little blood during your *menstrual period*. This is called menstruation. You will notice when it has started because there may be blood on your pants or in your *urine*. While you are menstruating you need to use *sanitary towels*, pads or *tampons* to soak up the *menstrual flow*. After menstruation, the endometrium starts to thicken again and the whole *menstrual cycle* repeats itself.

Many girls and women have no problems when they menstruate. Some get an ache or cramp-like pains in their lower *abdomen* before and during *menstruation*. If the pain is very bad (see dysmenorrhoea),

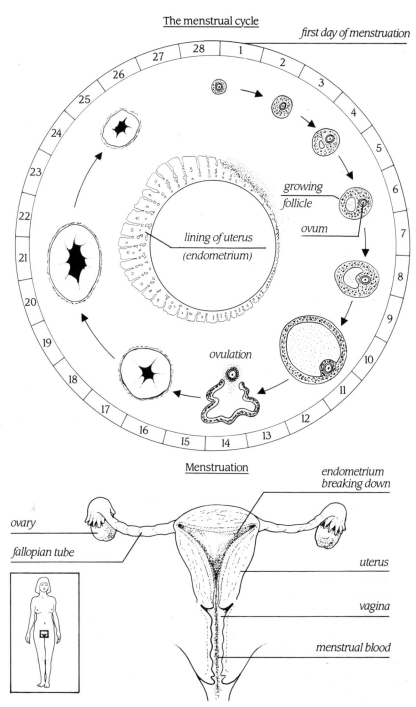

The menstrual cycle

first day of menstruation

growing follicle

ovum

lining of uterus (endometrium)

ovulation

Menstruation

endometrium breaking down

ovary

fallopian tube

uterus

vagina

menstrual blood

you may want to take painkillers or see your doctor about it. Some girls and women also get sore *breasts*, have headaches and feel tired, irritated or depressed before they menstruate (see *premenstrual syndrome*). Getting some exercise and taking care over what you eat can help if you have these kinds of problems. If they are very bad, you should see your doctor.

There is no need to change anything about the way you live when you are menstruating. There are many stories about what you can and can't do during your menstrual period – you mustn't wash your hair, have a bath, do sports etc. Although it is true that some religious and cultural groups have strict rules about what menstruating girls and women can and can't do, most girls and women can carry on as normal.

midwife A nurse who specialises in *pregnancy* and *birth*.

milk See *breastfeeding*.

mini-pill Some people use this to mean *progestogen-only pill*.

miscarriage (MISS-ca-rij) A *pregnancy* which ends before the 28th week. Doctors sometimes call a miscarriage a 'spontaneous abortion'. If a woman has a miscarriage, her baby usually dies, although sometimes it can be saved by a special care unit in a hospital. Early miscarriages (before the 12th week of pregnancy) are very common. About one in six pregnancies ends like this. Early miscarriages usually happen because there is something wrong with the baby. Later miscarriages (after the 12th week) are less common. They may happen if the woman's *placenta* is not working properly or if she has a weak *cervix* which opens too early (see *labour*). A miscarriage is hardly ever caused by the woman doing something wrong. Having a miscarriage can make you feel sad, angry and guilty. It is important to grieve over the loss of the unborn baby. This takes time. But if a woman has a miscarriage it doesn't mean she can't have another baby. Many women who have a miscarriage go on to have a successful pregnancy next time.

missionary position A way of having *sexual intercourse* in which the man lies on top of the woman so that they are facing each other.

to **molest** (mo-LEST) To annoy, disturb or attack someone, especially in a *sexual* way.

M

monogamous (mer-NOG-a-mus) Being married to one person at a time (see *monogamy*). This word can also be used to describe a *relationship* between two people who are sexually *faithful* to each other but not necessarily married to each other.

monogamy (mer-NOG-a-mi) Being married to one person at a time. All *marriages* have to be *monogamous* in the UK by law.

mons pubis (MONZ PEW-biss) The slightly raised fatty mound in a girl or woman which cushions and protects the *pubic bone* beneath it (see the drawing on page 115). In girls who have reached *puberty* and women, the mons pubis is covered with *pubic hair*. Also called the mons veneris.

mons veneris See *mons pubis*.

moods *Adolescence* is a time of growth and change. Having moods, or feeling up one minute and down the next, is all part of this change. Your moods usually settle down as you get older and start to get used to your adult body and feelings.

moral (MO-rul) This word means something which is in line with the morals or acceptable behaviour of society or of a group (see also *immoral*).

morning-after pill A method of *contraception* for women. The morning-after pill is for <u>emergency use only</u>. If a woman has *sexual intercourse* without using any contraception or if she thinks the *contraceptive* she or her *partner* used might not have worked (for example, if a *condom* split), she should go to see her doctor or a *family planning clinic* as soon as possible. The doctor may decide to give her the morning-after pill. If it is taken within three days of *unprotected sex*, it usually stops *pregnancy*. The morning-after pill should not be used regularly because it can upset your *menstrual cycle* and your *hormone* levels. See *contraception*.

morning sickness Feeling or being sick during *pregnancy*. Although it is called 'morning' sickness some *pregnant* women feel sick all day. Not all pregnant women get morning sickness. Women that do usually find that it disappears around the 12th to 14th week of pregnancy.

mucus method A less reliable version of the sympto-thermal method of *contraception*. See *natural methods* and *contraception*.

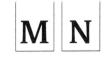

multiple birth When a woman gives birth to more than one baby at a time. This could be *twins* (two babies at the same time), triplets (three), quads (four), quins (five), sextuplets (six) etc.

N

naked (NAY-ked) Without clothes on.

natural childbirth When a woman has her baby without pain relief.

natural methods The aim of natural methods of *contraception* is to prevent *pregnancy* without using any *contraceptive* (such as a *condom*, *diaphragm* or *IUD*). To avoid pregnancy in this way, couples either do not have *sexual intercourse* at certain times of the month or the man does not *ejaculate* inside the woman's *vagina*. Couples using the rhythm method (or 'safe period') avoid sexual intercourse when they think the woman is at her most *fertile* (around *ovulation*). But this is not very reliable because it is difficult for the woman to know exactly when she is ovulating and there is no really safe time when a woman can be sure she will not get *pregnant*.

The most reliable way of working out when a woman is ovulating involves the woman checking daily for changes in her *cervical mucus* and body temperature. This is called the sympto-thermal method or 'double check' method. But it can take up to a year to learn this method and you need help from a specially trained teacher. Some couples try to avoid pregnancy by coitus interruptus (withdrawal). This involves the man taking his *penis* out of the woman's vagina before he ejaculates. But it is not a reliable method of contraception because *sperm* can leak into the woman's vagina at any point during sexual intercourse. The man may also not be able to stop himself from ejaculating while his penis is inside the woman's vagina.

navel (NAY-vul) The dimple in your *abdomen* which shows where your *umbilical cord* joined you to your mother before you were born

Some people call their navel their belly button.

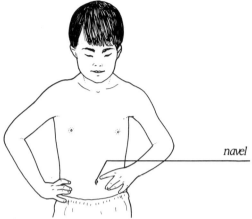

navel

neck of the womb Another expression for *cervix*.

necking You may find that some people don't like this word. It means *kissing*.

nipple (NI-pul) The nipple is at the centre of the *areola* (see the drawing on page 18). During *puberty*, a girl's breasts develop and the nipples grow too. Nipples can stick out, lie flat or turn inwards. In both men and women, tiny muscles underneath the nipple and the areola respond to cold, touch and *sexual arousal* and make the nipple hard and *erect*. If a woman is *breastfeeding* her baby, the *breast milk* flows out through tiny holes in the nipple.

nocturnal emission (nok-TER-nul i-MI-shun) When *semen* leaks out of an *adolescent* boy's *penis* while he is asleep. Also called a wet dream. If this happens to you, you may wake up and find a small amount of semen coming out of your penis. Or you may wake up in the morning and find a small amount of semen on your pyjamas or sheets. When the semen dries it can stain the sheets, but the stain should come out in the wash. Nocturnal emissions happen while you are dreaming, even if you are not dreaming about *sex*. They are a sign that your *reproductive organs* are developing and they can happen quite often during *puberty*. But don't worry if you don't have them – that's normal too.

NSU Stands for non-specific urethritis. A *sexually transmitted infection*. See the table on pages 93 to 96 and *sexually transmitted infection*.

nude Another word for *naked*.

nuts You may find that some people don't like this word. It means *testes*.

nymphomaniac (nim-fo-MAY-nee-ak) A woman who has very strong or frequent *sexual desire*. Some people use this word when a woman is clear about when she wants or needs *sex* because her openness makes them feel uncomfortable and they disapprove of her.

O

obstetrician (ob-ster-TRI-shun) A doctor who specialises in *pregnancy* and *birth*. An obstetrician works with a team of *midwives*, nurses and other doctors to provide *pregnant* women with *antenatal care* and to *deliver* their babies.

oestrogen (EE-strer-jun) One of the *female sex hormones* produced by the *ovaries* (see the drawing on page 44). The other sex hormone is *progesterone*. When a girl reaches *puberty*, her ovaries start to produce more oestrogen. This makes her *vagina* and other *reproductive organs*, her *breasts* and her *pelvis* start to grow. It also makes her *endometrium* start to thicken each month in case an *ovum* is *fertilised*. All these changes are a sign that the girl is turning into a young woman (see *puberty*) and that she is different from boys and men.

offspring Another word for children. You (and your brothers and sisters if you have any) are your parents' offspring.

to be 'on' Some people use this to mean having a *menstrual period*.

oral contraceptive (OR-ul) Another word for the *contraceptive* pill (either the *combined pill* or the *progestogen-only pill*).

oral sex (OR-ul) Using your mouth and tongue to *kiss*, lick or suck your *partner's genitals*. Both women and men can become *sexually aroused* and have *orgasms* in this way. When a woman has her genitals kissed, licked or sucked by someone, it is called cunnilingus. When a man has his *penis* kissed, licked or sucked by someone, it is called fellatio. A woman cannot get *pregnant* from getting *semen* in her mouth during oral sex. However, some *sexually* transmitted infections can be passed on through oral sex. There is a very small risk of catching *HIV* through oral sex if your partner is HIV-infected. See *HIV.*

organ (OR-gun) Any part of the body which keeps the body working, such as your eyes, your heart, your stomach or your lungs. See *reproductive organs.*

orgasm (OR-gaz-um) The peak of *sexual* excitement. You can have an orgasm either by having *sexual intercourse* with someone or by *masturbating.* To have an orgasm you need to be *sexually aroused.* Your *clitoris* or *penis* needs to be rubbed and *stimulated* until the feelings of pleasure and sexual tension become very strong. At orgasm this tension is suddenly released. This can send waves of intense pleasure through your whole body. When a man has an orgasm, *semen* spurts out of his penis (see *ejaculation*). Women do not ejaculate. Some women can have several orgasms, one after the other (this is called a multiple orgasm). Orgasms can be quiet like a sigh or very strong. They can be just a physical feeling or they can fill your whole body and mind. Most people feel very relaxed after they have had an orgasm and some people feel very sleepy. Two people who are having sexual intercourse or masturbating together may have their orgasms at the same time or one of them may have an orgasm before the other. Sometimes one of them may not have an orgasm at all. This does not necessarily mean that the other person has not pleased them or is not good at *having sex.* You can still enjoy sex without having an orgasm.

orgy (OR-ji) Can mean a group of people getting together to *have sex.* Most people do not have sex like this.

os (OSS) The opening of the *cervix.* When a girl or woman is having her *menstrual period, menstrual blood* passes through the os on its way out of the *uterus* into the *vagina.* During *pregnancy,* a mucus plug fills the os and seals off the uterus so that the unborn baby stays inside.

outer labia See *labia.*

ova (O-va) Plural of *ovum* (one ovum, two or more ova).

ovaries Plural of *ovary* (one ovary, two ovaries).

ovary (O-va-ri) Part of the *female reproductive system* (see the drawing on page 115). Girls and women have two ovaries, one on each side of the *uterus*. They are attached to the uterus by fibres. They are oval in shape and about 4cm (1½in) long by about 1¼cm (½in) wide. In girls who have reached *puberty* and in women, the ovaries take it in turns to release an *ovum* each month (see *ovulation*) and to produce the female *sex hormones* (see *oestrogen* and *progesterone*) which are responsible for some of the changes which take place during the *menstrual cycle*. During puberty these hormones also make a girl's *reproductive organs* grow and develop. The ovaries stop releasing *ova* after the *menopause*.

oviduct (O-vi-dukt) Another word for *fallopian tube*.

ovulate See *ovulation*.

ovulation (ov-you-LAY-shun) The release of a *mature ovum* by an *ovary*. Usually only one ovum is released but occasionally two or more *ova* are released at the same time. Ovulation is part of the *menstrual cycle*. Each month, a *hormone* called *Follicle Stimulating Hormone (FSH)* makes between 10 and 20 *follicles* in one of the *ovaries* start to grow and develop. Each follicle contains an ovum. All the ova start to mature in the ovary but usually only one ovum becomes fully grown or mature. This ovum moves towards the surface of the ovary. At ovulation, the surface of the ovary bursts open and the

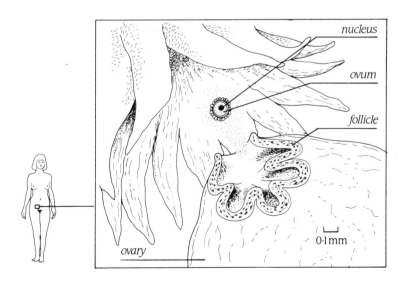

nucleus

ovum

follicle

0·1mm

ovary

ovum floats out towards the *fallopian tube*. Ovulation usually happens about 14 days before a girl's or woman's next *menstrual*

c

period, although not all women ovulate every month. Some women notice ovulation as a slight twinge or cramp in the lower *abdomen*. They may also notice a clear jelly-like *discharge* from their *vagina* and a feeling of increased vaginal wetness before and during ovulation. A woman is most *fertile* around ovulation so if she doesn't want to start a baby she needs to avoid *unprotected sexual intercourse* around this time or use a reliable method of *contraception*.

ovum (O-vum) The *female sex cell* (or egg cell). An ovum is so small (about 0.15mm across) that it can't be seen without a microscope. In girls who have reached *puberty* and in women, the *ovaries* take it in turns to release an ovum each month (see *ovulation*). The ovum travels down the *fallopian tube* and if it meets a man's *sperm* and is *fertilised* by it (see *fertilisation*), it lodges itself in the woman's *uterus* and starts to develop into a baby. Sometimes a fertilised ovum starts to develop before it gets to the uterus (see *ectopic pregnancy*). If it is not fertilised, it passes out of the woman's *vagina* in her *vaginal fluid*. Girls are born with about 400,000 *ova* stored in their ovaries. Only about 300–500 are released during a woman's *fertile* years (between puberty and the *menopause*). The remaining ova disintegrate (break into pieces).

P

pad See *sanitary towel*.

paedophile (PEE-der-fyle) A person (usually a man) who is sexually attracted to children. It is against the law for an adult to have any form of *sexual contact* with a child. See also *incest* and *sexual abuse*.

painful periods See *dysmenorrhea*.

partner (PART-ner) Someone you do something with. Some people use the word partner to mean the person they are going out with, married to, or living with. If you have a *sexual relationship* with someone, they can also be called your partner or sexual partner.

passion (PASH-un) A very strong feeling of *love* or *desire* for someone. This word can also mean a sudden outburst of anger or a strong feeling of sadness.

paternal (pat-ERN-ul) This word is used to describe something which is a feature of a father (as in 'paternal *love*' for a child).

pee You may find that some people don't like this word. It means *urine*. To pee means to pass urine.

peeping tom Some people use this to mean *voyeur*.

pelvic The area within your *pelvis* is called your pelvic area.

pelvic inflammatory disease (PID) (PEL-vik in-FLAM-er-tri di-ZEEZ) An infection in a woman's *fallopian tubes* and sometimes also in her *uterus* or *ovaries*. Pelvic inflammatory disease can be caused by *chlamydia* or certain other *sexually transmitted infections*. Other causes include *childbirth, miscarriage, abortion* or having an *IUD* fitted. If you have PID, you may have a swollen *abdomen*, more painful or irregular *menstrual periods*, a burning pain when you pass *urine*, pain or bleeding after *sexual intercourse* and a general feeling of being unwell. It is important to find out early on if you have PID so you can get an antibiotic to clear it up. If it is not treated or it is treated too late, it can make you *infertile* and leave you in permanent pain. You can get advice and treatment from your doctor or a *Special Clinic*.

pelvis (PEL-viss) A basin-shaped circle of bone where your hips are. The pelvis is the link between the bones in the bottom of your

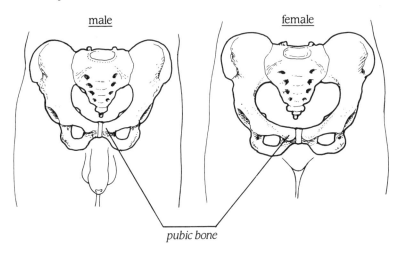

male

female

pubic bone

spine and the bones of your legs. The pelvis protects the *bladder* and *rectum* and in girls and women it also protects the *uterus*. During *puberty,* a girl's pelvis begins to widen. This is so that if she has a baby later on, there will be room for the baby to pass through the pelvis on its way out of the uterus and down the *vagina.*

penetrative sexual intercourse (PEN-a-trer-tiv) When a man's *penis* goes inside (or penetrates) another person's body during *sexual intercourse.* If he is having penetrative *sex* with a woman, his penis goes into her *vagina.* If he is having penetrative sex with a man, his penis goes into the other man's *rectum* during *anal intercourse.* You can get – or pass on – a *sexually transmitted infection* through penetrative sexual intercourse. If a woman has penetrative sexual intercourse without using *contraception,* she may get *pregnant.* The drawing on page 89 shows a man and a woman having penetrative sexual intercourse.

penis (PEE-niss) Part of the *male reproductive system* (see the drawing on page 114). Also used to pass *urine.* The penis is made up of a long *shaft* and a sensitive tip (called the *glans*). The glans has an opening in it. This is the opening of the *urethra.* Two types of *body fluids* can come out of this opening – urine and *semen.* Most of the time, your penis is soft, limp and not very big. But if you are *sexually aroused,* blood flows into your penis and it becomes hard and *erect.* If you have an *orgasm,* a small amount of semen spurts out of the hole in the tip of your penis (see *ejaculation*). It is impossible to pass urine and ejaculate at the same time. Many boys and men worry about the size of their penis. Your penis can look very small when it is limp. But when it is erect it is probably about the same size as everyone else's. In any case, the size of your penis makes no difference to your sexual enjoyment. If you are having a *sexual relationship* you can use a *condom* as a method of *contraception.* You can also use a condom to protect yourself against *sexually transmitted infections.* Unroll the condom onto your erect penis before *penetrative sexual intercourse* begins. If you notice an unusual *discharge* from your penis, it may be a sign of an infection and you should see your doctor or go to a *Special Clinic.*

perineum (per-in-EE-um) The area between a girl's or woman's *labia* and her *anus* (see the drawing on page 115). When a woman has a baby, her perineum has to stretch until it is very thin. It might even tear or have to be cut to let the baby through (see *episiotomy*).

period (PEER-i-od) See *menstrual period.*

personal hygiene (PER-ser-nul HY-jeen) Keeping your body clean. This is especially important during and after *puberty* because you sweat more and are more likely to get *BO.* Your sebaceous *glands* also produce more *sebum* (see *spots* and *acne*). Try to make sure your *hair,* teeth and nails are clean and that you wash your body regularly, especially your *genital* area and under your arms.

pervert (PER-vert) Someone who likes unusual *sexual activities* which would shock or offend most people.

pessary (PESS-a-ri) A soft tablet containing medicine which a girl or woman puts into her *vagina.* The tablet dissolves, releasing the medicine into her body. If you have *thrush,* you may be given pessaries by your doctor to treat it. You can also get *spermicides* in pessary form.

pethidine (PETH-i-din) A drug given to some women during *labour* to relieve pain.

petting (PET-ing) *Kissing* and cuddling. See also *heavy petting.*

phallus (FALL-us) Another word for *penis.* People may describe something as 'phallic' if its shape reminds them of the shape of a penis.

PID Stands for *pelvic inflammatory disease.*

piles Some people use this word to mean *haemorrhoids.*

the pill Some people use this word to mean the contraceptive pill. See *combined pill* and *progestogen-only pill.*

pimp Someone (usually a man) who sets a *prostitute* up in business. The pimp usually keeps a lot of the money which the prostitute earns.

piss This word may shock or offend some people. It means *urine.* To piss means to pass urine.

pituitary gland (pit-YEW-i-tri) The main *endocrine gland.* The pituitary gland is attached to the base of the brain (see the drawing on page 44). It is about the size of a grape. It controls the other endocrine glands, including the *ovaries* in girls who have reached *puberty* and in women and the *testes* in boys who have reached puberty and in men. When puberty begins, the pituitary gland

P

starts to produce certain *hormones* in greater quantities. These include growth hormone, which makes *adolescent* girls and boys grow, and *Follicle Stimulating Hormone (FSH)* and *Luteinizing Hormone (LH)*, which control a girl's or woman's *menstrual cycle*.

placenta (pla-SEN-ter) An *organ* inside a *pregnant* woman's *uterus* which supplies her unborn baby with the food and oxygen it needs to grow and develop (see the drawing on page 72). One side of the placenta is fixed to the wall of the woman's uterus. The *umbilical cord* comes out of the other side and goes into the unborn baby's *navel*. An unborn baby does not eat and breathe like we do. Instead, food and oxygen pass from the mother's blood through the placenta and down the umbilical cord to the baby. Waste from the baby passes back through the cord and placenta and into the mother's blood. *Antibodies*, which help the baby fight infections once it is born, can also pass through the placenta from the mother to the baby. So can harmful things like alcohol, drugs and nicotine from cigarettes. This is why it is best for pregnant women not to smoke, drink alcohol or take drugs.

planned parenthood When a couple make sure that each baby they have is a planned and wanted baby. They may do this by using *contraception* when they have *sexual intercourse* but do not want to start a baby.

platonic (pla-TON-ik) A platonic friendship does not involve *sex*.

to **play with yourself** Some people use this to mean to *masturbate*.

polygamy (pol-IG-a-mi) Being married to more than one person at the same time. Polygamy is against the law in the UK.

porn Short for *pornography.*

pornography (por-NOG-ra-fi) *Erotic* books, magazines, photographs, videos or films. Pornography shocks and offends many people. It often goes far beyond what most people think is okay. It may show *sex* with violence or sex with children. Many people disapprove of pornography because it doesn't show women and men as people with real feelings. In this way, pornography may prevent some men and women from having an equal and healthy *sexual relationship*. Other people think that some types of pornography are all right because they help us enjoy sex and find

70

out what we think is sexually exciting. In the UK, there is no law about pornography. There is, however, a law about 'obscene publications' which includes most pornography. An obscene publication is anything which is 'likely to deprave or corrupt' someone who sees or hears it. Having obscene materials for your own use is not against the law. Showing or lending these obscene materials to anyone else is against the law.

postnatal (POST-nay-tul) After the *birth* of a baby.

postnatal care (POST-nay-tul) Healthcare of a mother and her new baby by her doctor and health visitor to make sure that she and her baby are both fit and well and that the baby is growing and developing. A woman who has had a baby should have a *postnatal* check-up by her doctor about six weeks after the baby is born.

postnatal depression (POST-nay-tul) Feeling very miserable and depressed after the birth of your baby. Postnatal depression is not the same as the *baby blues*. It is much worse and it feels as though it will never go away. It happens when a new mother's *hormones* get out of balance. A mother with postnatal depression badly needs help from her health visitor or doctor. Talking to her *partner*, friends and relatives may also help her get through this difficult time.

the **pox** This word may shock or offend some people. It means *syphilis*.

pregnancy (PREG-nan-si) The time during which a woman has a baby developing and growing inside her *uterus*. Pregnancy starts when a *fertilised ovum* (see *fertilisation*) sinks into the *endometrium* in the woman's uterus (see *implantation*). Doctors and *midwives* do not time pregnancy from fertilisation but from the first day of a woman's last *menstrual period*. On this timing, pregnancy lasts for 40 weeks. But a pregnancy can be shorter or longer than this depending on whether the baby is early or late.

You can get more information about how the baby grows and develops during pregnancy from books about pregnancy and *birth*.

Doctors often divide pregnancy into three *trimesters*, each lasting for three months. During the first trimester, the woman can feel very tired and may have *morning sickness*. While the baby is developing and growing inside her, her body is changing too. Her *breasts* get larger and may hurt, she probably has more *vaginal discharge* and

These drawings show what the unborn baby looks like as it develops and grows inside the woman's uterus during pregnancy.

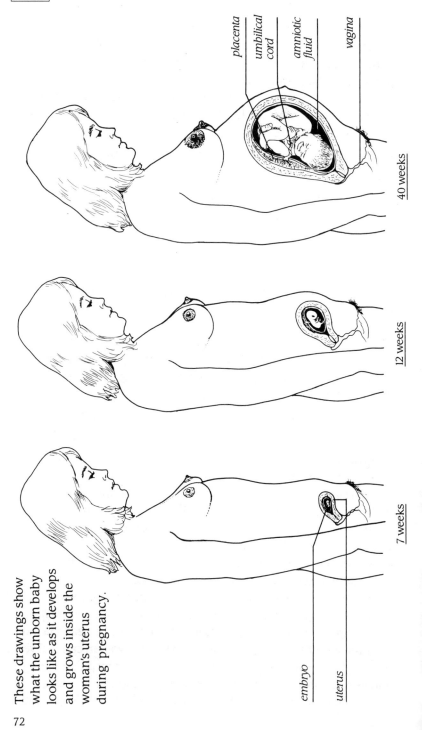

7 weeks

12 weeks

40 weeks

embryo

uterus

placenta

umbilical cord

amniotic fluid

vagina

needs to pass *urine* more often. She can also have a strange taste in her mouth and may go off, or have a craving for, certain foods. But by the end of the first trimester, the *fetus* is fully formed and many women start to 'bloom' – they look and feel really well. They may feel happy and excited about being *pregnant*. But most women also have days when they worry or are fed up with being pregnant.

If you are having a *sexual relationship* and don't want to get pregnant, you need to use some form of *contraception*. The different methods of contraception are listed on page 24. Some people think that a woman will not get pregnant if she has *sexual intercourse* standing up, passes urine straight after *sex*, has sexual intercourse during her menstrual period, or doesn't have an *orgasm*, or if the man takes his *penis* out of her *vagina* before he *ejaculates*. Don't listen to these stories – they are <u>not true</u>. Any of these ways of *having sex* can lead to pregnancy.

If you have had *unprotected sexual intercourse* and you think you might be pregnant, the first sign will probably be that your menstrual period doesn't come (although there are also other reasons for this happening – see *menstrual cycle*). If you think you could be pregnant, you should have a *pregnancy test* to tell you whether you are pregnant or not. You can arrange to have a test through your doctor, *family planning clinic* or a chemist. If the test says you are pregnant and you don't want to be, you must get help as soon as you can (see *abortion* and *adoption*). If you are pregnant and you are happy about it, the doctor will arrange for your *antenatal care* and the *birth* of your baby.

Most pregnancies end with the birth of a baby (see *labour*). But as many as one in six ends in *miscarriage*. And a few pregnancies sadly end with the death of the baby (a *stillbirth*).

pregnancy test A test to see if you are *pregnant* or not. Pregnancy tests work by seeing if there is a certain *hormone* in your *urine*. You can arrange to have a test through your doctor or *family planning clinic* or a chemist. Sometimes you have to pay for a test. You will need a sample of urine (if possible, from the first time you pass urine in the morning) in a clean, soap-free container such as a small jar. To be sure, you need to wait to do the test until two weeks after the first day of your missed *menstrual period*. If the test result is positive, you are almost certainly pregnant. If the test result is negative and you still haven't had your menstrual period a week later, you should have another test. You can also buy pregnancy

P

testing kits from the chemist for testing yourself at home. Home tests are quicker but they are expensive and must be used carefully. If you are eight weeks pregnant or more, your doctor can tell that you are pregnant by doing an *internal examination*.

pregnant (PREG-nant) A word used to describe a woman who is expecting a baby. See *fertilisation* and *pregnancy.*

premarital sex (pree-MA-ri-tul) *Having sex* with someone before you are married to them.

premature baby (PREM-a-chore) A baby born before the 37th week of *pregnancy* (pregnancy is expected to last for 40 weeks). Premature babies may need special medical care during the first few days or weeks of their lives, but they usually grow into normal, healthy babies. In some hospitals, babies born after only 26 or even 24 weeks of pregnancy have a chance of surviving.

premature ejaculation (PREM-a-chore i-jak-u-LAY-shun) When a man *ejaculates* sooner than he expects to or wants to.

premenstrual syndrome (PMS) (pree-MEN-strew-ul SIN-drome) When a girl or woman has the same problems every time she has her *menstrual period*. The problems usually start a week or two before *menstruation*. They vary from woman to woman but include things like depression, anxiety, mood swings, headaches, feeling dizzy, putting on weight, feeling bloated, sore *breasts*, and a craving for starchy and sweet things. The problems usually go away after her menstrual period has started and then come back again before her next one starts. PMS can sometimes be helped by changing the kind of food you eat, taking certain vitamins and minerals and getting regular exercise. If you have PMS and it is so bad that you feel you can't live your life normally, you should see your doctor. PMS is also called PMT or premenstrual tension.

premenstrual tension (PMT) See *premenstrual syndrome.*

prepuce (PREE-pewss) Another word for the *foreskin* of a boy's or man's *penis* or for the fold of skin or hood which usually covers a girl's or woman's *clitoris.*

prick This word may shock or offend some people. It means *penis.*

primary sexual characteristic See *sexual characteristic.*

private parts Some people use this to mean their *genitals*. Women may also use it to mean their *breasts*. Your private parts are the parts that are covered when you wear a bikini or swimming

Emergency contraception

If you have had sex without using contraception or think your method might have failed there are two emergency methods you can use.

- **Emergency pills** – must be started up to three days (72 hours) after sex. They are more effective the earlier they are started after sex.
- **An IUD** – must be fitted up to five days after sex.

Sexually transmitted infections

Male and female condoms can help protect against sexually transmitted infections. Male latex condoms should carry the BSI Kitemark (BS EN 600) and European CE mark. Diaphragms and caps may also protect against some sexually transmitted infections.

How fpa can help you

fpa's nationwide Contraceptive Education Service (CES) Helpline is open Monday to Friday and provides:

- confidential information and advice on contraception and sexual and reproductive health
- details of family planning clinics, sexual health clinics and other sexual health services
- a wide range of leaflets

fpa UK
2-12 Pentonville Road,
London N1 9FP
Phone 020 7837 4044
9am to 7pm

fpa Northern Ireland
113 University Street,
Belfast BT7 1HP
Phone 028 90 325 488
Derry 028 71 260 016
9am to 5pm

fpa Cymru
Ground Floor
Riverside House
31 Cathedral Road,
Cardiff CF11 9HB
Phone 0845 6001213
9am to 5pm

fpa Scotland
Unit 10
Firhill Business Centre
76 Firhill Road,
Glasgow G20 7BA
Phone 0141 576 5088
9am to 5pm

Ask fpa for a free copy of the following leaflets:

- Your guide to contraception (all methods)
- The progestogen-only pill
- Injections and implants
- The IUD
- The IUS
- Male and female condoms
- Diaphragms and caps
- Natural family planning
- Male and female sterilisation
- Emergency contraception
- After you've had your baby
- A guide to family planning services

A final word

This leaflet can only give you basic information about the combined pill. The information is based on the evidence and medical opinion available at the time this leaflet was printed. Different people may give you different advice on certain points.

Remember – *contact your doctor or a family planning clinic if you are worried or unsure about anything.*

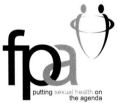

Registered charity number 250187.

Supported by the Department of Health, the Health Education Board for Scotland, the Health Promotion Division of the National Assembly for Wales and the Health Promotion Agency for Northern Ireland.

COC 02/00.

trunks. If you are *masturbating* or having a *sexual relationship* with someone, touching, *kissing* or stroking your own or your *partner's* private parts can give you good feelings and make you feel *sexually aroused*. But if someone you are not having a sexual relationship with wants to touch your private parts or wants you to touch theirs, find an adult you can trust and tell them what has happened. It's your body and no-one should touch you in a way or in a place that makes you feel uncomfortable (see also *sexual abuse* and *incest*).

progesterone (pro-JEST-a-rone) One of the *female sex hormones* produced by the *ovaries* (see the drawing on page 44). The other sex hormone is *oestrogen*. When a girl reaches *puberty,* her ovaries start to produce more progesterone. This makes her *endometrium* soft and spongy during the second half of each *menstrual cycle* so that if an *ovum* is *fertilised* it can sink into the endometrium and grow and develop into a baby. When a woman is *pregnant*, progesterone makes the muscles of the *uterus* more stretchy and softens the ligaments in the *pelvis* so it can get bigger to let the baby through when it is born. It also prepares the woman's *breasts* to produce *breast milk* once the baby is born.

progestogen (pro-JEST-a-jen) An artificial form of *progesterone.*

progestogen-only pill (pro-JEST-a-jen) A method of *contraception* for women. Also called the mini-pill because it only contains *progestogen* (the *combined pill* contains *oestrogen* <u>and</u> progestogen). The progestogen-only pill works in two ways. It makes the woman's *cervical mucus* thicker so that the man's *sperm* cannot easily swim through it and into the woman's *uterus*. And it makes it harder for a *fertilised ovum* to attach itself to the *endometrium*. It is very good at preventing *pregnancy* but you have to take it at exactly the same time each day or it may not work. Most women find that the progestogen only pill doesn't give them headaches, sore *breasts* or make them feel sick or put on weight, as the combined pill can do. But it can make their *menstrual periods* irregular, with bleeding at odd times during their *menstrual cycle* or no bleeding at all. You have to get the progestogen-only pill from your doctor or *family planning clinic* and you need to have regular check-ups. See *contraception.*

promiscuity See *promiscuous.*

promiscuous (pro-MISS-kew-us) A word used to describe someone who has a casual attitude towards *sex* and who may have

P

sexual intercourse with several different people over a short space of time.

prophylactic Another word for *condom*.

prostate gland (PROSS-tate) Part of the *male reproductive system* (see the drawing on page 114). The prostate *gland* surrounds the male *urethra*. It is about the size of a golf ball. It produces a fluid which helps *sperm* to make swimming movements and also helps to stop acid in the *urine* from damaging sperm. This fluid mixes with sperm as they go down the man's urethra and out of his *penis* when he *ejaculates* during *sexual intercourse* or *masturbation*.

prostitute (PROSS-ti-tewt) A person who *has sex* with someone for money.

prude (PROOD) Someone who finds bodies and *sex* embarrassing and doesn't like thinking or talking about them. Someone might call you a prude if, for example, you refuse to take off your clothes in front of them or look at *sexy* pictures with them. But it's your body and you shouldn't do anything you don't feel right about.

puberty (PEW-ber-ti) The time of life when you change from being a girl to being a woman or from being a boy to being a man. During puberty the appearance and shape of your face and body change and your *reproductive organs* and *genitals* grow and develop. Your feelings and *emotions* also change during puberty – see *adolescence*. Puberty is caused by *hormones*. It starts in your brain where the *hypothalamus* triggers the *pituitary gland* to start to produce hormones. These hormones cause changes in the *ovaries* in girls and the *testes* in boys. In a girl, the ovaries start to release an *ovum* each month. They also produce the *female sex hormones, oestrogen* and *progesterone*. In a boy, the testes start to produce *sperm*. They also produce the *male sex hormone, testosterone*. These hormones help the reproductive organs and genitals to continue to develop and also cause many of the changes listed below. After puberty, you are physically and sexually *mature*.

How girls change during puberty
- Your body grows (see *growth spurt*).
- Your *breasts* develop.
- *Pubic hair* grows around your genitals.
- *Hair* grows under your arms and you may grow more hair on your arms, legs and face.

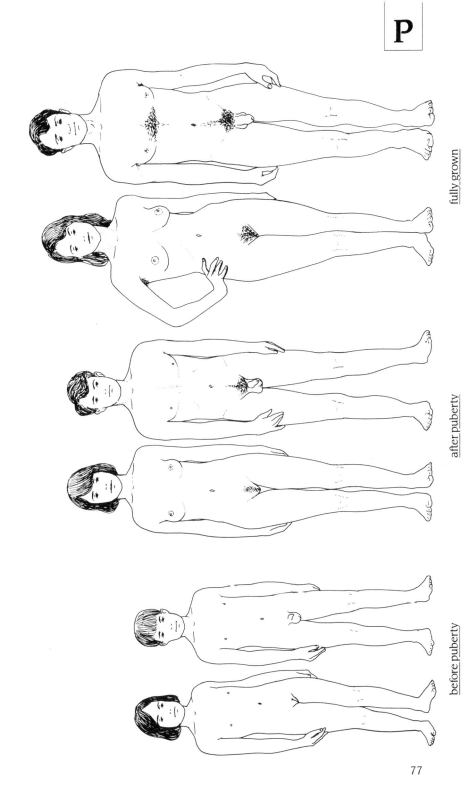

P

fully grown

after puberty

before puberty

77

- You have your first *menstrual period* (see *menstrual cycle* and *menstruation*).
- Your *pelvis* widens, giving you wider hips.
- Your body becomes more rounded.
- You sweat more, especially around your genitals and under your arms (see *personal hygiene*).
- *Sebum* may get thicker and block the pores in your skin, causing *spots* or *acne*.
- Your face changes shape and your forehead, jaw and nose become more prominent.
- Your voice gets a bit deeper (see *voice changes*).
- Your muscles get bigger and change shape.
- Your *labia* get bigger and darker and the outer labia grow hair (see *pubic hair*).
- Your *clitoris* grows and becomes more sensitive.
- Your *ovaries* start to release an ovum each month (see *ovulation*).
- Your *uterus* grows and builds up its lining (see *endometrium*) each month.
- Your *vagina* grows and produces more *vaginal fluid* (you may feel this as wetness around your genitals).

How boys change during puberty
- Your *testes* get bigger and start to produce *sperm*.
- Your *scrotum* gets darker and changes texture.
- Your *penis* grows and becomes more sensitive.
- You have more *erections*.
- You may have *nocturnal emissions* ('wet dreams').
- *Pubic hair* grows around your genitals. You may also have a line of hair growing from your *genital* area to your *navel*.
- *Hair* grows under your arms and on your face.
- You may also grow more body hair.
- Your body grows (see *growth spurt*).
- Your shoulders grow wider than your hips.
- You sweat more, especially around your genitals and under your arms (see *personal hygiene*).
- *Sebum* may get thicker and block the pores in your skin, causing *spots* or *acne*.
- Your face changes shape with your forehead and jaw getting longer.
- Your voice gets deeper (see *voice changes*).
- Your muscles get bigger and change shape.

These changes don't happen overnight. They can start any time from about age nine and can finish any time up to about age 18. A common age for girls to start puberty is 11 and a common age for boys is 13 but we are all different. This means you may have a friend who is the same age as you who has finished developing before your body has even started to change. If you are one of the first or last ones to start, you may feel embarrassed and get teased by the others. But don't worry – everyone's body develops and matures in the end.

You can get more information about what happens to your body during puberty by looking up the words that are written in italics (like this: *pubic hair*) in this dictionary. Also see the drawings on page 77.

pubes You may find that some people don't like this word. It means *pubic hair.*

pubic bone (PEW-bik) The bone at the front of your *pelvis* (see the drawing on page 67).

pubic hair (PEW-bik) The hair which grows around your *genitals* during *puberty* (see the drawings on pages 114 and 115). When it first grows, it is quite soft, but after puberty it becomes coarser and curly. Don't worry if your pubic hair is a different colour from the hair on your head – this is quite common.

pubic lice (PEW-bik) A *sexually transmitted infection*. See the table on pages 93 to 96 and *sexually transmitted infection*.

pudendum (pew-DEN-dum) The *genital* area. This word is especially used for the *female* genital area.

Q

queer You may find that some people don't like this word. It is sometimes used to describe a *lesbian* or a *homosexual*.

R

randy (RAN-di) Some people use this to describe a person who is keen to *have sex*. Can also mean *sexually aroused*.

rape When a man forces another person (usually a woman) to have *penetrative sexual intercourse* with him against their will. (If you have to do something 'against your will' it means you are forced to do something you don't want to do.) A man who rapes someone is called a rapist. Rape is a horrible crime. It is usually violent and very frightening for the person being raped. Not all rapists are strangers in dark alleys – they may know the person they rape. There are many different reasons why a man rapes. It might be because he has problems with his own *relationships* or *sex life* which make him feel angry and aggressive. A rape is <u>very rarely</u> caused by anything the girl or woman has done. If you have been raped, you should try to tell a friend or an adult you trust straightaway. If you decide to report the rape to the police, you should do so as soon as possible. Don't wash your hair, have a bath, tidy yourself up or change your clothes because you may destroy evidence against the man, such as his fingerprints, blood, hair or *semen*. Take someone with you to the police station if you can. You can also ring your local rape crisis centre for help and support. You can get their number by ringing the London Rape Crisis Centre on 071 837 1600.

rectum (REK-tum) The end of the digestive system, where waste is stored before it passes out of your *anus* when you go to the toilet (see the drawings on pages 114 and 115). Some people call the rectum the back passage. In *anal intercourse*, a man puts his *penis* through another person's anus and into their rectum. You can get *HIV* if an HIV-infected man has anal intercourse with you without using a condom (see *HIV*).

relationship (ri-LAY-shun-ship) When two people have regular contact or a connection of some kind. Having a relationship can also mean being more involved, such as going out together, being married or living together. It can be hard work having a relationship with someone. You may not always see things in the same way and you may get on each other's nerves sometimes. But having a relationship can also help you to grow and understand yourself and others better and make you happy. A *sexual relationship* is a relationship which involves *sexual contact*.

releasing factor See *hypothalamus*.

rent boy Some people use this to mean *male prostitute*.

reproduction (ree-pro-DUK-shun) The act or process by which new life is created. In human beings, reproduction takes place when a man and a woman have *sexual intercourse* and his *sperm fertilises* her *ovum*.

reproductive organs (ree-pro-DUK-tiv OR-ganz) The parts of the body which are responsible for *reproduction*. The reproductive *organs* make up the *reproductive system* (see the drawings on pages 114 and 115).

reproductive system (ree-pro-DUK-tiv SISS-tem) The parts of the body which are needed to start a baby. The *female* and *male* reproductive systems are different (see the drawings on pages 114 and 115). The female reproductive system includes these *reproductive organs: ovaries, fallopian tubes, uterus, cervix* and *vagina*. The male reproductive system includes these *reproductive organs: testes, epididymis, vas deferens, seminal vesicles, prostate gland, urethra* and *penis*. You can get more information about these reproductive organs by looking up the words that are written in italics (like this: *testes*) in this dictionary.

rhythm method See *natural methods*.

romance (RO-manss) A *love* affair which can be short and full of *passion* or last a lifetime. In a romance, the person you love means more to you than anything else in the world. You feel warm and tender when you think about them. You like being with them. And you take time and trouble to show them how special they are to you. For example, there may be a special place that you go to only with them. You might play music together which reminds you of how and when you met. In books and films, a romance often involves a handsome young man falling in love with a beautiful young woman and living happily ever after. Nothing else matters apart from their love for each other which is strong enough to overcome all difficulties. Real life is not always that simple. We are not all good looking and we do not always meet the perfect *partner* and stay with them for ever. But if romance comes our way, most of us can enjoy feeling special, making someone else feel special and putting everyday cares and worries to one side, even if it's only for a short time.

rubber Some people use this word instead of *condom*.

rubella (roo-BEL-a) A virus which many children get. Some people call it German measles. It is fairly harmless if a child gets rubella but if a *pregnant* woman gets it, particularly in the first three months of her *pregnancy*, it can damage her unborn baby. For this reason many girls are now given a vaccination against rubella. This usually happens when you are about 13. If a woman is planning to have a baby, she should have a blood test first to see whether she needs a rubella vaccination or not.

S

sadist (SAY-dist) Someone who enjoys hurting other people. A sadist finds it sexually exciting to hurt their *sexual partner*. Most people do not enjoy *sex* with pain.

safe period See *natural methods*.

safer sex *Sexual contact* where the risk of passing on *HIV* or other *sexually transmitted infections* is reduced. This can mean avoiding *penetrative sexual intercourse* so that infected *semen*, blood or *vaginal fluid* does not get into the other person's body, or, if you do decide to have penetrative sexual intercourse, making sure that a *condom* is used every time. Safer sex also means other activities where the man's *penis* does not go inside the other person's body. These include *kissing*, stroking, touching, massage, body rubbing (or frottage) and *masturbating* alone or with a *partner*.

sanitary towel (ST) (SAN-it-ri) A cotton pad which a girl or woman can use during her *menstrual period* to soak up the *menstrual blood* as it leaves her *vagina*. The sanitary towel goes inside your pants. Many STs have a sticky strip on the back which you stick to your pants. There are different thicknesses so that you can buy the ones that suit you best. For example, if your menstrual periods are light, you only need a thin ST. Or you may need a thick one at the beginning of your menstrual period when it is heavier and a thin one at the end when it is lighter. You should change the ST every few hours. This is because menstrual blood starts to smell once it has left your body and has come into contact with bacteria in the air. Most STs can't be flushed away down the toilet. To get rid of them, you can wrap them in a tissue or in toilet paper and put them in the dustbin. In public toilets, there are usually special paper bags and bins or incinerators for disposing of STs. You can also buy much smaller pant liners or pads which can be used at the end of your menstrual period when it is very light. These can usually be flushed away down the toilet. Another way of soaking up menstrual blood is to use a *tampon*.

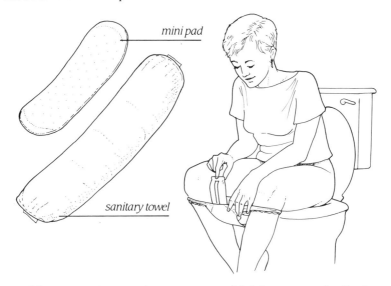

mini pad

sanitary towel

scabies (SKAY-beez) Tiny creatures which burrow under the top layers of the skin and make you itch very badly. The itching is often worse at night. You may also have red, raised bumps on the skin, particularly between the fingers, on or under the *breasts*, around the waist or wrists, and on the *genitals* or *buttocks*. Scabies is usually passed on by close contact with an infected person. You can get rid of it by treating your whole body with a special lotion which you can buy from the chemist. Some people also wash their bedclothes, towels and flannels in very hot water to avoid getting scabies again, although the risk of infection in this way is very small. Scabies can be passed on through *sexual contact* with an infected person but this is rare.

to **screw** This word may shock or offend some people. It means to have *sexual intercourse*.

scrotal sac See *scrotum*.

S

scrotum (SKRO-tum) The loose pouch of wrinkled skin which hangs down behind a boy's or man's *penis* and which contains the *testes* (see the drawing on page 114). Also called the scrotal sac. The testes can only produce *sperm* at a temperature of 35°C, which is 2°C cooler than the temperature inside our bodies. They hang in the scrotum outside the body so that they can stay at this cooler temperature. If they get too cold, the skin of the scrotum shrinks, drawing the testes up towards the body for warmth. If they get too hot, the scrotum drops slightly so that the testes can cool down.

sebum (SEE-bum) An oily substance which is produced by the sebaceous *glands* in your skin. Sebum helps to keep your *hair* and skin waterproof and your skin supple. During *puberty*, the sebaceous glands start to produce more sebum. This can give some *adolescents* greasy hair and *spots*. See also *acne* and *personal hygiene*.

second stage of labour See *labour.*

secondary sexual characteristic See *sexual characteristic.*

self-abuse People sometimes use this expression instead of *masturbation*, particularly if they don't approve of people masturbating.

semen (SEE-men) A liquid which comes out of the tip of the *penis* of a boy who has reached *puberty* or of a man when he *ejaculates*. Semen is a milky, sticky liquid. It is made up of *seminal fluid*, fluid from the *prostate gland*, and millions of *sperm*. About a teaspoonful of semen comes out each time a boy or man ejaculates. There are about 400 million sperm in this much semen. During puberty, some boys wake up at night to find semen coming out of their penis. Or they may wake up in the morning and find semen on their pyjamas or sheets. This probably means that they have had a *nocturnal emission* ('wet dream'). Because semen contains sperm, a woman can get *pregnant* if she has *unprotected sexual intercourse* with a man. Men can also pass on *HIV* and other *sexually transmitted infections* through their semen, although wearing a *condom* can help to prevent this.

seminal duct Another term for *vas deferens.*

seminal fluid (SEM-in-ul FLEW-id) Fluid produced by the *seminal vesicles* of boys who have reached *puberty* and of men. This fluid mixes with *sperm* and other substances from the *prostate gland* to make *semen*. Semen comes out of a boy's or man's *penis* when he *ejaculates*.

seminal vesicle (SEM-in-ul VEEZ-i-kul) Part of the *male reproductive system* (see the drawing on page 114). There are two seminal vesicles, one going into each *vas deferens*. They are small *glands* which produce *seminal fluid*.

sex Your gender – whether you are *male* or *female*. Some people also use this word to mean *sexual intercourse*.

sex cell Some people use this to mean an *ovum* or a *sperm*.

sex drive Another term for *libido*.

sex hormone (SEX HOR-mone) The sex hormones control *sexual* growth and development during *puberty*. The main *female* sex hormones are called *oestrogen* and *progesterone*. The *male* sex hormone is called *testosterone*. During *puberty* the *ovaries* and the *testes* produce sex hormones in greater quantities. This makes the *reproductive organs* and the *genitals* grow and develop. The sex hormones are also responsible for many of the other physical changes which take place during puberty. Low levels of the female sex hormones are found in boys and men and low levels of testosterone are found in girls and women. After puberty, the female sex hormones are involved in a girl's or woman's *menstrual cycle*.

sex life Your sex life is the *sexual* side of your life.

sex organs Some people use this to mean the *genitals* and/or *reproductive organs*. For more information about the sex organs <u>outside</u> your body, look up *genital* in this dictionary. For more information about the sex organs <u>inside</u> your body, look up *reproductive system* in this dictionary.

sexist (SEX-ist) A sexist person thinks that women's and men's lives are determined by what *sex* they are. This can be very limiting for both men and women because it assumes that all men will behave in a certain way and that all women will behave in a different way. In fact, people are different anyway – it doesn't matter what sex they are. For example, not all boys and men like woodwork and football. Not all girls and women like cooking and want to have children.

sexual (SEX-you-ul) A word used to describe something to do with *sex* or a person's sex.

S

sexual abuse (SEX-you-ul a-BEWSS) When a person does something sexual to you against your will or forces you to do sexual things with them. Sexual abuse usually happens within a family (see *incest*). For example, children (boys and girls) may be sexually abused by their father, stepfather, mother's boyfriend, grandfather, uncle, a close family friend or a brother. Boys are sometimes sexually abused by women but this is less common.

If you are being sexually abused, the man might touch your *breasts, vagina* or *anus* (if you are a girl) or your *penis* or anus (if you are a boy). He might make you undress while he watches, or you may be forced to stroke his penis or put it in your mouth. He might also make you have *sexual intercourse* with him.

Sometimes the man might make you do these things by threatening to hurt you. He might persuade you to let him do what he wants by telling you how special you are and how much he needs you and your body. He might trick you by telling you that what he is doing is normal. He might get you to promise to keep his 'little secret' or say that if you tell anyone he will go to prison. If he is your father or your mother's boyfriend, he might say your mother doesn't *love* him but you do and this is how you can show you love him. He might even say that if you don't let him do what he wants, he will hurt someone you love such as your mother or little sister or brother.

But you have to remember that <u>there is no excuse for what he is doing. It is totally wrong and it is against the law</u>. He is older and stronger than you and he is taking advantage of his power over you. So don't blame yourself for what is happening or has happened. <u>It isn't your fault</u>.

If you are being, or have been, sexually abused, telling someone may be the hardest thing you ever have to do. But you must try to tell someone. Choose who you tell carefully. Find someone you know you can trust. It may be better to choose someone outside your family. Telling a friend can be okay, but you will also need to find an adult who can help you.

When you tell someone, this is what should happen. You should feel that they are listening to you and that they understand and believe what you are saying. They should say to you that you were right to tell them. They may have to tell someone else what you have told them. But they shouldn't leave you without letting you know what they are going to do and what might happen next. If you tell one person and they don't help, <u>don't give up</u>. Try to find someone else who will believe and help you.

If you are being, or have been, sexually abused, <u>you are not alone</u>. On pages 119 and 120 is a list of organisations which can give you help and advice. If you can't find anyone to tell, telephone or write to one of these organisations.

sexual activity (SEX-you-ul) Any activity which involves *sexual contact*. *Sexual intercourse, oral sex* and *deep kissing* are all sexual activities.

sexual arousal (SEX-you-ul a-ROWZ-ul) A feeling of being sexually excited or aroused. Many things can make you sexually aroused. It can be something you see, hear, smell or touch. Or it can be a *sexual fantasy*, a *sexy* picture or book or a dream. *Masturbating* can also make you feel sexually aroused. *Kissing*, cuddling, touching, stroking or *caressing* your own or your *partner's* body, particularly the *genital* area and especially the *clitoris* or *penis*, are all ways of increasing sexual excitement. If you become sexually aroused, your body goes through a series of changes which are sometimes called your sexual response. Not everyone goes through the same changes, but this is the basic pattern:

Male	Female
More blood flows into his *penis*.	More blood flows into her *vulva* and *clitoris*.
His *testes* swell and draw up closer to his body.	Her *genital* area swells and feels full.
His penis becomes hard and *erect*.	Her clitoris becomes hard and *erect* and comes out from under its hood. She starts to produce more *vaginal fluid* and her *labia* begin to feel quite wet.
His body feels alive to touch, his muscles start to tense up and contract, his heart starts to beat faster and his breathing becomes faster and shallower.	Her body feels alive to touch, her muscles start to tense up and contract, her heart starts to beat faster and her breathing becomes faster and shallower.
His *nipples* may become erect and more sensitive.	Her *nipples* may become erect and more sensitive.

Male	Female
	Her *breasts* may swell and a flush or rash may appear on her skin. When she is fully aroused, her clitoris goes back under its hood.
If he has an *orgasm*, sexual tension is released (see *orgasm*).	If she has an *orgasm*, sexual tension is released (see *orgasm*).
If sexual arousal stops or if no orgasm is reached, the blood slowly flows away from the *genitals* back into the rest of his body, his penis goes limp and his body relaxes.	If sexual arousal stops or if no orgasm is reached, the blood slowly flows away from the *genitals* back into the rest of her body, the swelling goes down and her body relaxes.

sexual characteristic (SEX-you-ul ka-rak-ter-ISS-tik) A physical feature which distinguishes a boy or man from a girl or woman. The primary sexual characteristics are the *reproductive organs*. These are the parts of the body which are involved in starting a baby. They grow and develop during *puberty* and are different in men and women. The secondary sexual characteristics also grow and develop during puberty. They are not involved in starting a baby but they act as a signal that men and women are different and can lead to *sexual* attraction. They include *breasts*, body and facial *hair, voice changes* and changes in body shape.

sexual contact (SEX-you-ul) *Kissing*, touching or stroking another person's body in a *sexual* way. It can also mean *sexual intercourse*.

sexual discrimination (SEX-you-ul) When someone is treated less favourably than someone else because of their *gender* or *sex*.

sexual harassment (SEX-you-ul ha-RASS-ment) Repeated and unwanted sexual comments, looks, suggestions or physical contact which make you feel uncomfortable or which you find offensive. If someone your own age, a teacher, or someone you work with is doing this, you need to tell someone. Find someone you can trust. It might be someone in your family. If you are being harassed at school, you might be able to tell a form tutor or a head of year. If it is happening at work, you might be able to tell a supervisor or manager. Tell them what is happening. You will need to give as much detail as you can. If the person you tell doesn't believe or help you, contact the Equal Opportunities Commission to see what else you can do. Their address is on page 119. See also *sexual abuse*.

sexual intercourse (SEX-you-ul IN-ter-korss) When a man slides his *erect penis* into a woman's *vagina*. This is sometimes called vaginal intercourse. Two men can have sexual intercourse when one man slides his erect penis through the other man's *anus* and into his *rectum*. This is called *anal intercourse*. Having sexual intercourse is also called having sex.

When a man has sexual intercourse his penis must be erect. For this to happen, he needs to be *sexually aroused*. It is possible for a woman to have sexual intercourse without being aroused but she may not enjoy it and it may be uncomfortable because the inside of her vagina will be too dry. See *sexual arousal* and *foreplay*.

This drawing shows one way in which a man and a woman can have sexual intercourse.

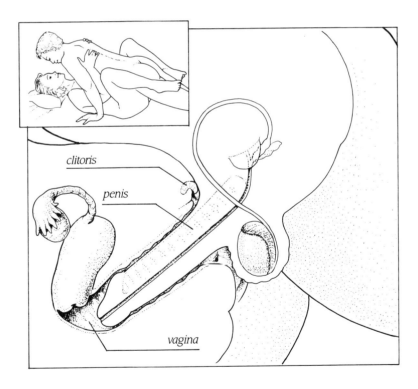

clitoris

penis

vagina

S

When a man and a woman have sexual intercourse, the man slides his penis inside the woman's vagina. The couple then move rhythmically together so that his penis slides up and down inside her vagina. This builds up sexual excitement until one or both of them has an *orgasm*. When a man has an orgasm, *semen* spurts out of his penis. This is called *ejaculation*. If they are not using *contraception*, the woman may get *pregnant*. After sexual intercourse, the man's penis goes soft and he takes it out of the woman's vagina. The woman's body slowly returns to how it was before she was sexually aroused. If the man and woman want to have sexual intercourse again, they can as soon as the man's penis is erect. This will not happen immediately.

If two men are having a *sexual relationship*, they might decide to have anal intercourse. Although it is physically possible for a man and a woman to have anal intercourse, it is against the law. See *anal intercourse*.

Many people with a disability can enjoy sex. It's true that pain, tiredness and medicines can lower your *sex drive*. And some disabilities reduce feeling in the *genitals* and make it difficult to have an orgasm. But if you have a disability, it doesn't mean that sex is not for you. It might mean though that you have to experiment to find ways of having sex which suit you, use extra lubrication (see *KY jelly*) and, if you need contraception, think carefully about which method is best for you. You could also contact the Association to Aid the Sexual and Personal Relationships of People with a Disability (SPOD) for help and advice. Their address is on page 119.

There are lots of reasons why people have sexual intercourse. They may want to show *love* for each other, and being physically close and giving each other pleasure is one way of doing this. A man and a woman may have sexual intercourse because they want to start a baby. Some people have sex just to find out what it is like or because of the pleasure it gives them.

How, where, how often and for how long you have sexual intercourse varies from person to person. Your sexual feelings and needs can change as you change, grow older, or perhaps change *sexual partner*. No-one can tell you what sexual intercourse will be like for you. This does not mean that you have to rush off and find out! If you have not had sexual intercourse, it may be because you are below the *age of consent*. Or you may be waiting until you get married. You may belong to a religious or cultural group that does not allow sex before *marriage*. Don't let the fact that your friends are (or say they are) already having sex push you into doing the same if you don't want to. It's your body and no-one has the right to have sexual intercourse with you unless you have decided that this is what you want. (If someone in your family or a close family friend is making you have sexual intercourse, it is important that you turn to page 86 and read what it says under *sexual abuse*.)

If you are thinking about having sexual intercourse with someone, there are other things to think about too. For example, if a man and a woman don't want to start a baby they need to think about contraception. You also need to make sure you don't get a *sexually transmitted infection* (see *sexually transmitted infection* and *HIV*).

The first time you have sex you may be a little nervous. Being worried, frightened or shy can make it hard to relax. You need to trust each other and to take time and trouble to make sure that both of you are sexually aroused before intercourse. For a woman, the first time she has sexual intercourse may be a little painful and she may bleed slightly if the man's penis breaks her *hymen*.

If you are already having sexual intercourse, make sure you talk to your *partner*. That way you can share the good feelings that you have for each other and find out what you like and don't like when you are having sex. Many couples go on having sex well into old age and will tell you that it gets better as you get older. Some people stay *celibate* all their lives and never have sexual intercourse with anyone. You don't have to have sex in the dark or in bed. You might want to be the person who suggests sex and takes the lead, or your partner might want to. You can make as much noise as you like providing you don't disturb other people. There is no right or wrong way to have sexual intercourse. You have to find out what is right for you and your partner and work at making sex a good experience for both of you.

sexual maturity See *maturity*.

sexual orientation (SEX-you-ul or-i-en-TAY-shun) Your sexual orientation is whether you are *bisexual, heterosexual, lesbian* or *homosexual*.

sexual partner See *partner*.

sexual relationship See *relationship*.

S

sexual response See *sexual arousal.*

sexuality (sex-you-AL-i-ti) Feelings about being *male* or *female* and how you deal with these feelings. Some people explore their sexuality through *sexual fantasy* or *masturbation.* Many people explore their sexuality through *sexual contact* and their *relationships* with other people.

sexually active (SEX-you-al-i AK-tiv) This term can be used to describe someone who has *sexual contact.*

sexually aroused See *sexual arousal.*

sexually transmitted infection (STI) A general term for any infection which you can get by having *sexual contact* with an infected person. Also called sexually transmitted disease (STD), venereal disease (VD) or genito-urinary infection. If you are not having sexual contact with anyone you don't need to worry about sexually transmitted infections. If you <u>are</u> having sexual contact with someone and either you or your *sexual partner* has had sexual contact with someone else in the past, one of you may have an STI. Sometimes there are obvious signs (or symptoms) that you have got an STI – see the symptoms listed in the table on the next four pages. But sometimes there are no clear signs or symptoms.

There are at least 25 different infections which can be passed on during *sex.* The most common ones are listed in the table. Most infections can affect both *males* and *females.* STIs affect the *genitals* or the parts of the body that *urine* passes through (the *bladder* and the *urethra*). They can also affect the mouth and throat if they are spread through *oral sex.* Most STIs can be treated and cured. A few can make you very ill if they are not treated. Some can make women *infertile.* If you think you or your sexual partner has an STI, you must go to a doctor or *Special Clinic* for treatment as soon as you can. (If a woman is *pregnant* she should tell her doctor before she is given treatment because the treatment may damage her unborn baby.)

If you are *having sex,* it makes sense to protect yourself against STIs. There are several things you can do:

1 Limit the number of people you have sex with. If you only have sex with one person and they have only ever had sex with you, you can't get an STI.
2 Don't have sex with someone who has an unusual *discharge* from their *penis* or *vagina* or whose *genital* area looks sore or blistered.
3 Use a *condom* or *diaphragm.*
4 Pass urine and wash your genital area after having sex.
5 Finally, tell your sexual partner if you have, or think you might have, an STI.

Name of STI	Cause	Symptoms	Treatment
chlamydia (kla-MI-dee-a)	A bacterium which you can get by *having sex* with someone who is infected.	Women: ● pain or a burning feeling when they pass *urine* ● a thin *vaginal discharge* and/or pain in the *abdomen* perhaps with a fever. (Many women have no symptoms until the infection has spread to the *fallopian tubes*.) Men: ● a burning feeling when they pass *urine* ● a *discharge* from the *penis*.	Antibiotics from your doctor or a *Special Clinic*. In women, chlamydia can lead to *pelvic inflammatory disease (PID)*. PID can make a woman *infertile*. So if you have had *sexual contact* with someone who has got chlamydia, you should go to your doctor or a *Special Clinic* straightaway.
cystitis (siss-TY-tiss)	Bacteria which you can get by *having sex*. But you can also get cystitis without *sexual contact*. For this reason, it is explained in the dictionary under 'c' for *cystitis*.		
genital herpes (JEN-i-tul HER-peez)	A virus which you can catch by *having sex* with someone who has an active infection.	● itching, tingling or aching in the *vulva*, *penis* or *testes* followed by: ● sores, usually on and around the *genital* area. Some women have sores on their *cervix* too but they cannot feel these. The sores change to watery blisters in a day or two and usually burst and heal themselves without treatment. While you have the sores, you may: ● feel pain when you pass *urine* ● feel as though you've got flu (headache, backache and high temperature).	There is no cure for genital herpes but there are remedies to make you feel more comfortable if you have it. Your doctor or *Special Clinic* might be able to help. The Herpes Association has a telephone helpline. Their telephone number is on page 119.

S

Name of STI	Cause	Symptoms	Treatment
genital warts (JEN-i-tul WARTZ)	A virus which you can catch by *having sex* with someone who is infected.	• fleshy growths or warts on the *genital* area. They may also grow in the *vagina, anus* or *cervix* where they cannot be easily seen.	Sometimes a special ointment is painted on the warts to get rid of them. There may be a link between genital warts and *cervical cancer*. Women who have had genital warts or whose *sexual partners* have genital warts should have regular *cervical smear tests*. If you think you have genital warts you should go to your doctor or a *Special Clinic*.
gonorrhoea (gon-o-REE-a)	A bacterium which you can get by *having sex* with an infected person.	60% of women and 10–15% of men who have gonorrhoea have no symptoms. Others have: • pain when passing *urine* • an unusual *discharge* from the *vagina* or a yellowish discharge from the *penis* • an itchy *anus* or a discharge from the anus • a sore throat if you have caught gonorrhoea through *oral sex*. Women may also have: • a fever or 'chill' • pain in the *abdomen* • painful joints (knees, wrists etc).	Antibiotics which you can get from your doctor or a *Special Clinic*. You need to have regular check-ups after you have finished the antibiotics to make sure the infection has been cleared up.

Name of STI	Cause	Symptoms	Treatment
hepatitis B (hep-a-TY-tiss BEE)	A virus which you can catch by *having sex* with someone who is infected. The virus is passed on from one person to another through infected *body fluids*.	Many people have no symptoms. Some people: • feel as though they've got flu and have a cough and sore throat • feel very tired and lose their appetite • have painful joints (knees, wrists etc). You may develop jaundice in which case: • your skin and the whites of your eyes turn yellowish • your *urine* turns darkish brown and your *faeces* become light and clay-coloured • you may have pain in your *abdomen*.	Plenty of rest and healthy food. Gradually your body returns to normal. But you may still be infectious for years and may need to think about *safer sex*. (There is a vaccine against hepatitis B but it is only given to people who are most likely to catch the virus such as health workers, *sexual partners* of infected people or people travelling to certain countries.)
HIV (human immuno-deficiency virus)	A virus which you can catch by *having sex* with someone who is infected. But you can also get HIV without *sexual contact*. For this reason, it is explained in the dictionary under 'h' for *HIV*.		
NSU (non-specific urethritis)	A bacterium which you can get by *having sex* with someone who is infected. Doctors do not always know which bacterium causes NSU (that's why it's called 'non-specific').	Urethritis means inflammation of the *urethra*. Symptoms include: • pain when passing *urine* • *discharge* from the *penis*.	Antibiotics which you can get from your doctor or a *Special Clinic*.
pubic lice (PEW-bik LICE)	Small lice (insects) in the *pubic hair* which can be spread by close body contact during sex.	• very itchy *genital* area • small eggs or nits (empty egg cases) attached to your *pubic hair*.	A special lotion which you put on your *genital* area. You can get it from a *Special Clinic*. Ordinary washing with soap and water will not kill the lice or get rid of the nits.

Name of STI	Cause	Symptoms	Treatment
scabies (SKAY-beez)	Scabies can be passed on through *sexual contact* with someone who is infected but this is rare. See *scabies* under 's' in this dictionary.		
syphilis (SI-fi-liss)	A bacterium which you can get by *having sex* with an infected person. Syphilis is not very common these days.	Stage 1: 1–2 weeks after infection • a painless sore on or near the *vagina* or *penis*. Stage 2: 2–6 weeks after infection • a rash on the body • you feel as though you've got flu (headache, sore throat, fever). Stage 3: years after infection Stage 3 is very rare because most people are cured before this stage. Symptoms are: • permanent damage to the heart, brain and other *organs*.	Can be cured with antibiotics which you can get from your doctor or a *Special Clinic*. You will need regular check-ups after you have finished the antibiotics to make sure the infection has been cleared up. Syphilis must be treated early. If it is left untreated, it can kill you.
thrush	A yeast infection which you can get by *having sex* with someone who is infected. But you can also get thrush without *sexual contact*. For this reason, it is explained in the dictionary under 't' for *thrush*.		
trichomoniasis (tri-ko-mo-NY-ay-siss)	A tiny organism or *cell* which affects the *vagina* and *urethra*. You can get trichomoniasis by *having sex* with someone who is infected.	Women: • yellow or white *discharge* from the *vagina* which is quite smelly • itchy vaginal area. Men: May have no symptoms so they may not know they have got it.	Special tablets which you can get from your doctor or a *Special Clinic*.

sexy (SEX-i) If you look sexy, some people might find you sexually attractive. Feeling sexy means feeling *sexually aroused*.

shaft The long part of a boy's or man's *penis* (see the drawing on page 114).

to shag This word may shock or offend some people. It means to have *sexual intercourse*.

shaving Removing unwanted *hair* with a razor. During *puberty*, boys start to grow hair around the chin, cheeks and top lip. If you

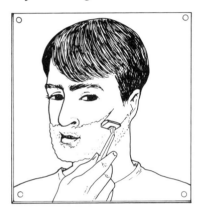 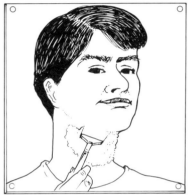

leave this hair, it eventually grows into a beard and moustache. If you decide you don't want to leave it, you can shave it off with an electric razor or with an ordinary razor using shaving soap (or shaving cream) and warm water. Start below one ear and work round to your chin, shaving downwards. Then do the other side of your face, your top lip and under your chin. For a closer shave, you can try shaving upwards. Splashing water or aftershave on your face after you have shaved can sting but it will help to close up the pores of your skin. Girls who have reached puberty and women should not shave off unwanted facial hair or stray hairs (see *hair*). Some women shave off the hair from their legs and from under their arms but there is no need to do this if you don't want to.

sheath Another word for *condom*.

short and curlies This expression may shock or offend some people. It means *pubic hair*.

'show' A sign that *labour* is beginning. It happens when the plug of mucus in the *cervix* comes away and passes out of the *vagina*.

S

Sometimes the 'show' doesn't happen until the woman is already in labour.

sibling Another word for brother or sister.

single parent A man or woman who is bringing up his or her child or children alone.

slag This word may shock or offend some people. It is used by some people to describe a girl or woman who *sleeps around*.

to **sleep around** To be *promiscuous* and not worry too much about who you *have sex* with.

to **sleep together** Some people use this instead of to have *sexual intercourse*.

to **sleep with someone** Some people use this instead of to have *sexual intercourse*.

slit This word may shock or offend some people. It means *vulva*.

S/M Stands for sado-masochism. See *sadist* and *masochist*.

smegma (SMEG-ma) A substance produced by *glands* under the *foreskin* of a boy's or man's *penis*. Smegma is a whitish waxy substance which helps the skin slide smoothly back over the tip of the penis when a boy or man has an *erection*. *Adolescent* boys and men who have not been *circumcised* should roll back their foreskin and wash regularly under it so that the smegma doesn't become smelly or infected.

snogging You may find that some people don't like this word. It means *deep kissing*.

sodomy Another word for *anal intercourse*.

to **solicit** (sol-ISS-it) To approach someone in a public place and offer to *have sex* with them in return for money.

Special Clinic A clinic where you can get treatment for *sexually transmitted infections* and other *genito-urinary infections*. Special Clinics are usually in main hospitals. For the address of the Special Clinic nearest to you, look in the phone book under 'Special Clinic', 'genito-urinary (GU) clinic', 'sexually transmitted disease' or 'venereal disease'. Treatment at Special Clinics is free and confidential and you don't need a letter from your doctor. See *sexually transmitted infection*.

speculum (SPEK-you-lum) A metal or plastic instrument which a doctor uses during an *internal examination*. It is put into the woman's *vagina* and opened slightly to hold the vaginal walls apart. It is also used when a *cervical smear test* is done.

sperm The *male sex cell.* A sperm looks a bit like a tadpole, with a head, a neck and a tail. It is so tiny (about 0.05mm long) that it can't be seen without a microscope. It is much smaller than the *female* sex cell (the *ovum*). In boys who have reached *puberty* and in men, sperm are produced in the *testes.* Up to 100 million sperm can

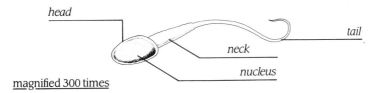

head

tail

neck

nucleus

magnified 300 times

mature in 24 hours. When a man *ejaculates*, about 400 million sperm are squeezed up the *vas deferens* where they mix with *seminal fluid* and other substances from the *prostate gland* to make *semen.* The semen then spurts out of the tip of the *penis.* 400 million may sound like a lot of sperm but they are so tiny that the semen wouldn't look any different if you took all the sperm out. If a man is having *unprotected sexual intercourse* with a woman, and his penis is inside her *vagina* when he ejaculates, the sperm can swim through the woman's *cervix* into her *uterus* and travel up her *fallopian tubes.* If a single sperm meets a mature ovum here and joins with it (see *fertilisation*), a baby starts. Only one sperm is needed to *fertilise* an ovum. As soon as this sperm gets through the outer layer of the ovum, a chemical change takes place which stops any other sperm from getting in. A boy or man only produces as much sperm as is needed. So if he is not ejaculating (because he is not *masturbating* or having sexual intercourse), the production of sperm slows down. During puberty, you may find that your body is producing sperm that you don't need. Some of this sperm may leak out of your penis while you are asleep (see *nocturnal emission*). This is a normal part of growing up. A man can go on producing sperm until well into old age, unlike women who stop releasing *ova* once they reach the *menopause.*

sperm duct Another term for *vas deferens.*

S

spermatozoon (sper-ma-ta-ZO-un) A medical word for a single *sperm*. Two or more sperm are called spermatozoa.

spermicide (SPER-mi-side) A substance which kills *sperm*. You can buy spermicide as a cream, jelly or foam or in *pessaries*. It is not a reliable method of *contraception* if it used on its own because you cannot be sure that all the sperm will come into contact with the spermicide. But using spermicide with a *diaphragm* or *condom* can make these methods of contraception more reliable and effective. Some condoms already have spermicide on them when you buy them. It says on the packet if they do.

sponge See *contraceptive sponge*.

spontaneous abortion See *miscarriage*.

spots Small raised bumps on the surface of the skin. Spots are very common during *adolescence*. This is because during *puberty*, sebaceous *glands* in your skin start to produce more *sebum*. Your *sex hormones* may then make the sebum thicken, causing it to block the pore. As the sebum comes into contact with the air, it turns black, causing what is known as a blackhead. Infection can start underneath the blackhead and cause a small red pimple filled with pus. It is very tempting to squeeze spots and pimples but this can make the infection worse. Spots are most common on your face, back, shoulders and *chest*. No-one likes having spots. But if you have spots, try not to hide away or you may miss out on life. You need to find a way of coping with your spots which works for you.

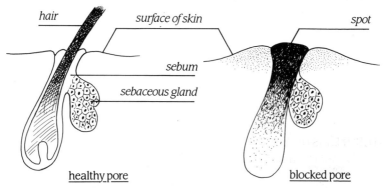

Some people stop using soap and switch to special lotions to wash their face with. Others try to cut down on fatty foods like chocolate and chips. If these methods make your spots better or make you feel better, carry on with them. Unfortunately, not everyone can get rid of their spots in this way. If you have lots of spots and they are infected and pus-filled, see *acne*.

spunk You may find that some people don't like this word. It means *semen*.

ST Stands for *sanitary towel*.

stages of labour See *labour*.

sterile (STE-ryle) Unable to start a baby. See *infertile*.

sterilisation (ste-ri-ly-ZAY-shun) A permanent method of *contraception* for both men and women. Sterilisation makes you *sterile* so you cannot start a baby. *Male* sterilisation is called vasectomy and involves closing off both of the *vas deferens*, so that *sperm* cannot travel into the man's *urethra* and out of his *penis*. After a man has been sterilised, and once his *semen* no longer contains sperm, he cannot make a woman *pregnant*. But he can still have *erections, ejaculate* and enjoy *sex* in the same ways that he did before he was sterilised. *Female* sterilisation involves closing off both *fallopian tubes* so that *ova* cannot travel into the *uterus*. This means that the woman cannot get *pregnant*. But she still has *menstrual periods* and she can enjoy *sex* in the same ways that she did before she was sterilised. Very occasionally, the sterilisation operation is not a success because the vas deferens or fallopian tubes rejoin. But this is very unusual and, generally speaking, you should think of sterilisation as a permanent method of contraception. It is only suitable for someone who is absolutely sure that they won't want any children (or any more children) and that they won't change their mind later. See *contraception*.

to **sterilise** See *sterilisation*.

STI Stands for *sexually transmitted infection*.

stillbirth (STIL-berth) When a baby is born dead. Some babies also die shortly after they are born. The Stillbirth and Neonatal Death Association can give parents help and counselling if their baby dies. Their address is on page 120.

to **stimulate** (STI-mew-late) To excite or make more active.

straight Some people use this word to mean *heterosexual*.

S T

to **suck off** Some people use this to mean to give someone an *orgasm* by sucking or licking their *genitals*. See *oral sex*.

suppository (ser-POZ-i-tri) A soft tablet containing medicine which you put inside your *rectum* or *vagina*. The tablet dissolves, releasing the medicine into your body.

sympto-thermal method See *natural methods*.

syphilis (SI-fi-liss) A *sexually transmitted infection*. See the table on pages 93 to 96 and *sexually transmitted infection*.

T

tampax (TAM-pax) This is a make of *tampon*. Some people use this word instead of tampon.

tampon (TAM-pon) A finger-shaped roll of cotton wool which a girl or woman can put into her *vagina* when she has a *menstrual period* to soak up the *menstrual flow*. There are different kinds of tampons. They are all wrapped in plastic or paper which you have to take off first. Some of them are inside a thin cardboard tube. To insert this kind of tampon, you gently push the cardboard tube into your vagina and with your finger push the tampon out of the tube into your vagina. You then pull the tube out of your vagina, leaving the tampon inside, and throw the cardboard tube away. Other tampons don't have a cardboard tube around them and you simply push them into your vagina with your finger. All tampons have a string at one end. You put the tampon in so that most of this string hangs down outside your vagina. You pull on the string when you want to take the tampon out.

Tampons come in different sizes. If you have not used a tampon before and want to try one, buy a packet of the smallest size and put a tampon in your vagina next time you have your menstrual period, following the instructions in the packet carefully. You will know when it is in properly because you won't be able to feel it at all. Putting a tampon in for the first time can hurt a little because it may stretch or break your *hymen*. (In some religious and cultural groups where it is important for unmarried women to have an unbroken

102

hymen, girls may be told not to use tampons.) Changing the tampon regularly is very important. You should change it when you get up in the morning, before you go to bed and usually two or three other times during the day. Don't forget to take the last one out when you finish your menstrual period. Wash your hands before and after you change the tampon. Some people prefer using a tampon to a *sanitary towel* or pad because you can't feel it when it is in properly, it can't be seen and you don't have to worry about smell. Tampons are also smaller to carry around and you can flush used ones down the toilet.

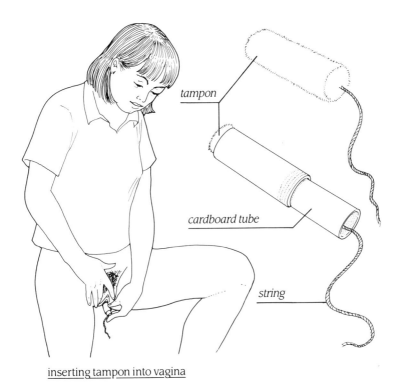

tampon

cardboard tube

string

inserting tampon into vagina

termination Another word for *abortion*.

test tube baby See *IVF.*

testes (TESS-teez) Plural of *testis* (one testis, two testes).

testicle (TESS-ti-kul) Another word for *testis.*

testicular self-examination (TSE) (tess-TIK-you-la) Checking your *testes* (or testicles) for unusual lumps or changes which could be a sign of cancer. McCormack Ltd produces a leaflet on testicular self-examination (their address is on page 119).

testis (TESS-tiss) Part of the *male reproductive system*. The two male *testes* hang down behind the *penis* (see the drawing on page 114). They are held in the *scrotum* and are about the size of small plums. The left testis usually hangs down lower than the right one. The testes produce the male *sex hormone, testosterone,* which causes the changes in a boy's body during *puberty.* Inside each testis are about 100m (325ft) of tiny coiled tubes. *Sperm* are made inside these tubes from puberty until well into old age. If a man or boy *ejaculates* during *masturbation* or *sexual intercourse,* replacement sperm are made in the testes.

testosterone (tess-TOSS-ter-oan) The *male sex hormone* which is produced by the *testes* (see the drawing on page 44). When a boy reaches *puberty,* testosterone makes his *genitals* grow and develop and causes *hair* to grow on his face and genitals and under his arms. It also makes him grow taller (see *growth spurt*), and makes his shoulders broader and his voice deeper. It may make him more aggressive. All these changes are a sign that the boy is turning into a young man (see *puberty*) and that he is different from girls and women.

third stage of labour See *labour.*

thrush An infection which affects the *vulva* or *vagina* in women and may affect the *penis* in men. It is caused by a yeast called candida albicans. We all have this yeast inside our bodies. Most of the time it doesn't cause any problems. But sometimes it gets out of control and causes infections, especially in women. Signs for a woman that she has got thrush include an itching around her vulva and a thick white *discharge* from her vagina. The vulva may also smell a little and it may hurt to pass *urine.* Signs for a man that he has got thrush include a sore and itchy *penis.* Thrush can start if you are on antibiotics. It can be triggered by using vaginal deodorants, washing your *genital* area with very perfumed soaps and wearing nylon pants or even tight jeans. *Pregnant* women often get thrush. Thrush can also be caused by *sexual contact.* Women who think they have thrush can try treating themselves by putting a *tampon* dipped in plain yoghurt into their vagina. If this doesn't work, they should see their doctor. They will probably be given *pessaries* and possibly a cream. These should stop the itching and clear up the infection. Men are usually given a cream.

time of the month Some people use this expression to mean *menstrual period*.

tits This word may shock or offend some people. It means *breasts*.

tool This word may shock or offend some people. It means *penis*.

to **toss off** This expression may shock or offend some people. It means to *masturbate*.

to **touch someone up** Some people use this to mean when you touch someone in a *sexual* way and they don't want you to. See *sexual abuse*.

toxic shock syndrome (TSS) A very rare but serious disease which women using *tampons* can get. You should not get TSS if you use tampons correctly.

transsexual (tran-SEX-you-ul) A person who feels very strongly that they were born with the body of one *sex* and the mind of the other. For example, a woman may have a *female* body but think and feel like a man. Transsexuals usually want to change sex and some do go on to have a sex change operation in hospital.

transvestite (tranz-VESS-tite) A person who likes wearing clothes of the opposite *sex*. For example, a man might like wearing dresses, make-up and wigs. A few transvestites dress like this because it makes them *sexually aroused*.

trichomoniasis (tri-ko-mo-NY-ay-siss) A *sexually transmitted infection*. See the table on pages 93 to 96 and *sexually transmitted infection*.

trimester (try-MESS-ta) This word means three months. Doctors often divide the nine months of *pregnancy* into three three-month periods and these are called trimesters.

triplets Three babies born from the same mother at the same time.

tubal ligation A method of *female sterilisation*.

tubal pregnancy Another term for *ectopic pregnancy*.

turn off Some people use this to describe something which stops them feeling *sexually aroused*.

T

turn on Some people use this to describe something which makes them feel *sexually aroused*.

twat This word may shock or offend some people. It means *vulva*.

twins Two babies born from the same mother at the same time. It is quite common to have twins. About one in every 100 *pregnant* women gives birth to twins. A woman is more likely to have twins if there are twins in her family. Non-identical twins are quite

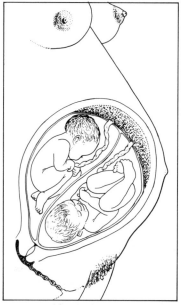
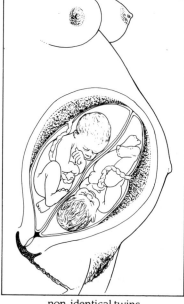

identical twins   non-identical twins

common. Non-identical means that the twins do not look exactly the same as each other. They can be a girl and a boy, two boys or two girls. You get non-identical twins when a woman's *ovary* releases two *ova* at the same time and they are both *fertilised* by *sperm*. Identical twins are much less common. Identical twins look almost exactly the same as each other. They are always both boys or both girls. You get identical twins when a fertilised *ovum* splits into two halves with each half containing exactly the same *DNA*. Siamese twins are very rare. You get Siamese twins when a fertilised ovum starts to separate into two halves but does not completely split. The two halves stay joined together and the babies are born attached to each other. A pregnant woman can find out if she is going to have twins when she has an *ultrasound scan*.

U

ultrasound scan (UL-tra-sound SKAN) A test which is carried out by a doctor on a *pregnant* woman to check the age and size of her unborn baby and to make sure it is developing properly. An ultrasound machine uses sound waves to create a picture of the unborn baby moving about inside its mother's *uterus*. You can see the picture on what looks like a television screen. Most pregnant women have at least one ultrasound scan during their *pregnancy*. Having an ultrasound scan doesn't hurt the mother or the baby.

umbilical cord (um-BI-li-kul KORD) The cord through which an unborn baby gets the food and oxygen it needs to grow and develop while it is inside its mother's *uterus* during *pregnancy* (see the drawing on page 72). An unborn baby does not eat and breathe like we do. Instead, food and oxygen pass from the mother's blood through the *placenta* and down the umbilical cord to the baby. Waste from the baby passes back through the cord and placenta and into the mother's blood. One end of the cord is attached to the baby. The other end is attached to the placenta. When the baby is born, the umbilical cord is clamped and cut. This does not hurt the baby or its mother. A little bit of cord is left attached to the baby. New skin forms under this bit of cord and after about a week, the cord drops off. The baby is left with a dimple where the cord was. This is its *navel*.

uncircumcised (un-SER-kum-sized) A man or boy who has not been circumcised. See *circumcision*.

underarm hair See *hair*.

unprotected sexual intercourse *Sexual intercourse* between a woman and a man without using any form of *contraception*, or between two men without using a *condom*.

urethra (you-REE-thra) A thin tube which carries *urine* from the *bladder* to the *urinary opening*. In girls and women, the urethra leads to a hole just in front of the *vagina*. In boys and men, the urethra runs down the middle of the *penis* to a hole at the tip of it. In boys who have reached *puberty* and in men, the urethra can also carry *semen* and is part of the *reproductive system*. If a man has an *orgasm*, semen comes down the urethra and out of his penis when

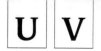

he *ejaculates*. It is impossible to pass urine and ejaculate at the same time. The *female* urethra is shorter than the *male* urethra. This means that girls and women can get infections of the bladder like *cystitis* more easily than boys and men.

urinary opening (YOU-rin-ri) The hole at the end of your *urethra* which *urine* comes out of (see the drawings on pages 114 and 115). In boys and men, the urinary opening is in the tip of their *penis*. In girls and women it is just in front of the *vagina*.

urine (YOU-rin) A *body fluid* which is stored in your *bladder* and passes out of your body when you go to the toilet. Urine comes out of a hole called your *urinary opening*. Urine is mainly made up of water and salts which your body doesn't need. Boys and men pass *urine* out of their *penis*.

uterine lining Some people use this instead of *endometrium*.

uterine tube Some people use this instead of *fallopian tube*.

uterus (YOU-ter-us) Part of the *female reproductive system* (see the drawing on page 115). Also called the womb. All girls are born with a uterus. During *puberty* it grows to about the size and shape of an upside down pear. Each month as part of the *menstrual cycle*, the lining of the uterus (the *endometrium*) thickens in case an *ovum* is *fertilised* by a *sperm* (see *fertilisation*). If the ovum is not fertilised, the thickened endometrium breaks down and passes out of the girl's or woman's *vagina* as her *menstrual period* (see *menstruation*). When a woman is *pregnant*, the uterus contains the unborn baby. It has to stretch a lot to make room for the baby to grow. By the time the baby is ready to be born, the uterus may be more than 50cm (20in) long from top to bottom. During *labour*, muscles in the uterus tighten and relax in order to pull the *cervix* open so that the baby can pass out of the uterus (see *contraction*). More contractions then help to push the baby through the vagina and out of the mother's body. After the baby is born, the uterus starts to return to its normal size.

V

vagina (va-JY-na) Part of the *female reproductive system*. The vagina is a muscular tube inside a girl's or woman's body which connects her *uterus* to the outside of her body (see the drawing on page 115). It is about 10cm (4in) long. The walls of the vagina are made up of soft folds of skin. If something goes into the vagina, such as a *tampon* or a man's *penis* during *sexual intercourse*, these folds stretch as it goes in. When a woman *gives birth* to a baby, the baby passes down through the vagina on its way out of the mother's body (although see *caesarian section*). The vagina has to stretch a lot for the baby to get through. The inside of the vagina can be dry or wet (see *vaginal fluid*).

vaginal discharge See *discharge*.

vaginal fluid (va-JY-nul FLEW-id) Fluid produced by the *glands* inside the *vagina* of girls who have reached *puberty* and of women. You may feel this as wetness on your pants. If you have not had your first *menstrual period* but have noticed some wetness, don't worry. This probably means that you will start to *menstruate* soon. Vaginal fluid keeps the vagina clean and healthy. It can be clear and watery or thick and white (on your pants it might look yellowish). Around the time of *ovulation*, there is more vaginal fluid and it becomes clearer and stretchier. The vagina also produces more fluid when a woman is *sexually aroused*. Different amounts of vaginal fluid are produced at different times. Drier times are before *puberty*, every month just after *menstruation*, when a woman is *breastfeeding* and after the *menopause*. Wetter times are when a woman is *sexually aroused*, around ovulation and during *pregnancy*. Vaginal fluid which looks or smells unusual can be a sign that you have an infection (see *discharge*).

vaginal intercourse See *sexual intercourse*.

vaginal lips See *labia*.

vaginal opening (va-JY-nul) The opening to the *vagina* (see the drawing on page 115) which may be partly covered by a thin membrane called a *hymen*. In girls who have reached *puberty* and in women, the *menstrual blood* comes out of this opening. During *penetrative sexual intercourse* between a man and a woman, the man puts his *penis* into the woman's vaginal opening. When a woman *gives birth*, the baby comes out of the opening. Although the opening is very small, it can stretch a lot.

vaginismus (va-ji-NIZ-mus) When the muscles in a woman's *vagina* tighten up during *penetrative sexual intercourse*, making it

V

difficult for the man's *penis* to get into the vagina. Vaginismus is quite rare. A woman who has this problem should see her doctor.

vaginitis (va-ji-NY-tiss) An infection of the *vagina*. If a woman has an unusual *discharge* from her vagina or if it hurts when she passes *urine*, she may have vaginitis and should see her doctor.

vas deferens (VAZ DEF-er-enz) Part of the *male reproductive system*. There are two vas deferens (see the drawing on page 114). They are muscular tubes, one coming out of each *testis*, which join the *urethra* as it leaves the *bladder*. They are about 40cm (16in) long and about as thick as a piece of string. When a man *ejaculates, sperm* are squeezed through these tubes and out of his *penis*.

vasectomy (va-SEK-to-mi) Another word for *male sterilisation*. See *sterilisation*.

VD Stands for *venereal disease*.

venereal disease (ver-NEER-i-ul) Nowadays most people use the term *sexually transmitted infection* instead of venereal disease.

vestibule (VESS-ti-bewl) Another name for the delicate area between the inner *labia* of girls and women. This includes the *urinary opening* and the *vaginal opening*.

viable (VY-er-bul) A word used to describe an unborn baby which would have a good chance of surviving if it was born *premature* or early. If a baby is born after 28 weeks of *pregnancy* it is said to be viable. Before 28 weeks, the baby is said to be not viable (even though babies born before 28 weeks can sometimes survive because of the special care they get in hospital).

virgin (VER-jin) Someone who has never had *sexual intercourse*. A virgin can be a *male* or a *female*. There is no way of telling whether a boy or man is a virgin. A broken *hymen* may be a sign that a girl or woman is not a virgin but a hymen can also be broken in other ways (see *hymen*). When you *have sex* for the first time, you are said to have lost your virginity.

virgin birth (VER-jin) When a woman who has never had *sexual intercourse* gives *birth* to a baby. This happens if a woman who is a virgin has *artificial insemination* or *IVF* and becomes *pregnant*. Virgin births are very unusual.

virile (VI-ryle) Some people use this word to describe someone who is very manly.

voice changes When your voice gets deeper during *puberty*. Both girls' and boys' voices get deeper as their larynx (or voice box) grows. In boys, it is usually called your voice breaking. Boys' voices get deeper than girls' because their voice boxes grow bigger. Your voice may change slowly or it may suddenly get deeper. Some boys find that they go through an in-between stage when their voice is breaking. Their voice may suddenly get very squeaky when they are talking. This happens when the muscles in the voice box go out of control for a moment. This stage can be embarrassing but it doesn't usually last long.

voyeur (voy-ER) Someone who is *sexually aroused* by watching people undressing or *having sex*.

vulva (VUL-ver) Another word for the *female genitals* (see the drawing on page 115). It is difficult to see your vulva properly without using a mirror. Many girls and women feel unsure about looking at or touching their vulva. But if you are familiar with your vulva it can help you understand your body and make you feel more confident about asking a doctor questions. If you look at your vulva in a mirror, you should be able to see your outer *labia*. After *puberty,* these will have *pubic hair* growing on them. If you gently separate your outer labia, you should be able to see your inner *labia, clitoris, urinary opening* and *vaginal opening.* Your vaginal opening may be covered by a thin layer of skin called a *hymen.* You can find out more about all these words which are written in italics (like this: *hymen*) by looking them up in this dictionary.

W

to **wank** You may find that some people don't like this word. It means to *masturbate*.

warts See *genital warts* in the table on pages 93 to 96 and *sexually transmitted infection.*

waters breaking See *amniotic fluid.*

wee Some people use this word to mean *urine.* To wee means to pass urine.

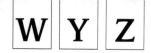

wet dream Some people use this instead of *nocturnal emission*.

whore (HOR) This word means *prostitute*. Some people use it to show that they disapprove of prostitutes.

willy You may find that some people don't like this word. It means *penis*.

withdrawal method See *natural methods*.

womb Another word for *uterus*.

Y

yeast infection See *thrush*.

Z

zits Some people use this word instead of *spots* or pimples. See also *acne*.

zygote Another word for a *fertilised ovum*.

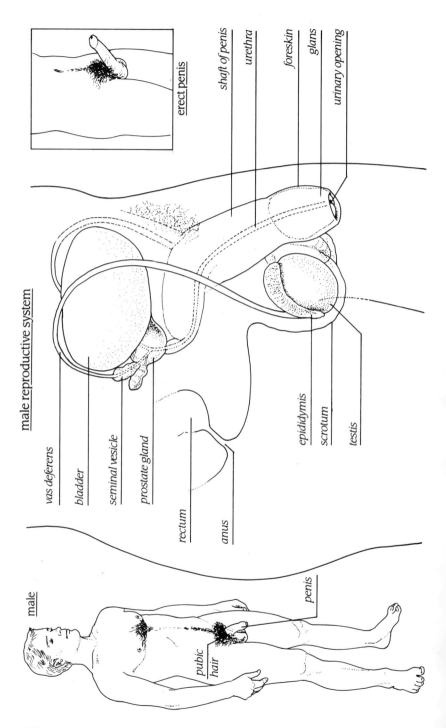

male reproductive system

erect penis

shaft of penis
urethra
foreskin
glans
urinary opening

vas deferens
bladder
seminal vesicle
prostate gland

rectum
anus

epididymis
scrotum
testis

male

penis

pubic hair

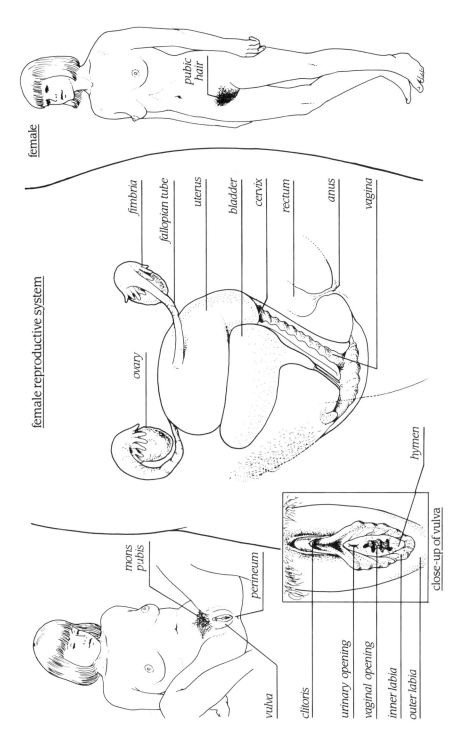

female

female reproductive system

fimbria
fallopian tube
uterus
bladder
cervix
rectum
anus
vagina

ovary

hymen

mons pubis

perineum

vulva
clitoris
urinary opening
vaginal opening
inner labia
outer labia

close-up of vulva

To parents, carers and anyone working with young people

If you are comfortable talking to young people about sex, the **LDA Sex Education Dictionary** is an ideal book to give to, or share with, any child or children in your care. But many people find it difficult to be open and honest with young people about sexual growth and development, personal relationships, pregnancy and birth. If you are embarrassed or unsure about any of these, read the statements and comments below. All the statements have been made by parents, carers, teachers or school governors. Each statement is followed by a comment which you might find helpful when you are trying to deal with your own feelings about young people and sex.

"My greatest worry is starting sex education with my child too early."
There's no such thing as too early. Personal and social development starts for children from the moment they're born. Children learn naturally about human interaction and social behaviour from the way they are held and talked to as babies, the love and attention they are given as they grow up, and the people who play with them, bath and dress them, teach them things and talk to them. They also learn by observing the way the people in their lives behave towards each other and how comfortable these people are with their own bodies. Unfortunately, not all the messages children receive as they grow up are clear or positive ones. You can help by filling in gaps, correcting misunderstandings, offering reassurance, commenting on experiences you have shared and answering questions. And the earlier you start this, the easier it is to grow with a child and adjust to their changing needs.

"I worry that if you tell young people about sex, they'll go off and try it."
The reverse appears to be true. Research suggests that sex education does not encourage early sexual activity. In fact, a recent study by the Guttmacher Institute in the USA indicated that the number of teenage pregnancies was considerably

lower in industrialised countries which have liberal attitudes towards sex, accessible contraceptive services for young people and effective formal and informal programmes of sex education.

"Not knowing about sex when I was young didn't do <u>me</u> any harm."
Not knowing things is okay for some people. But ignorance can leave others open to some of the more unpleasant consequences of sexual activity such as exploitation, sexual abuse, unwanted pregnancy and sexually transmitted infections. It can cause untold misery, for example, for girls who think that they are bleeding to death when their menstrual periods start, or for boys who think they have wet the bed when they have had a nocturnal emission. And ignorance about relationships and sexuality can take away a young person's choice – the choice to say no to sex if that is what they want to do.

"I want my child to learn about sex in a clear moral context."
The **LDA Sex Education Dictionary** aims to inform and reassure. Its moral context is that it encourages tolerance, understanding, communication and a caring, considerate and responsible attitude towards others. But it has not been written according to a specific moral code – it is for young people of all backgrounds, no matter what their colour, race, religion, social class, family grouping or sexual orientation. So if your religion or culture has a specific belief or code which you feel is not adequately covered in the dictionary, you may wish to make this clear to the child or children in your care.

To teachers

If you teach in a county, controlled or maintained special school, it is the duty of the governing body, under Section 18(2) of the Education (No 2) Act 1986, to consider whether sex education should form part of the secular curriculum and, where appropriate, to make and keep up to date a separate written statement with regard to the content and organisation of sex education within the school. At the time of writing, it was expected that the study of AIDS would become compulsory for all pupils aged 11 and over by the end of 1991.

The **LDA Sex Education Dictionary** should help you teach several aspects of sex education which have been formally included in the National Curriculum. At the time of publication, Old Attainment Target 3 (Processes of Life) in the document *Science in the National Curriculum* offers many relevant statements of attainment at different levels:

Level 1 Pupils should be able to name or label the external parts of the human body.

Level 2 Pupils should know that living things reproduce their own kind.

Level 3 Pupils should be able to describe the main stages in the human life cycle.

Level 4 Pupils should understand the process of reproduction in mammals.

Pupils should know about the factors which contribute to good health and body maintenance including the defence systems of the body.

Level 5 Pupils should understand the way in which microbes and lifestyle affect health.

Level 6 Pupils should know about the physical and emotional changes that take place during adolescence, and understand the need to have a responsible attitude to sexual behaviour.

Pupils should understand the processes of conception in human beings.

These will need to be checked against the New Attainment Targets as and when they are finalised. The document *Curriculum Guidance 5: Health Education* (National Curriculum Council, 1990) also recommends appropriate areas for study for sex education and for family life education at each of the key stages.

Useful addresses

Association to Aid the Sexual and Personal Relationships of People with a Disability (SPOD)
286 Camden Road
LONDON N7 0BJ
Tel: 071 607 8851

Provides advice, information, support and counselling to young people with a disability.

British Agencies for Adoption and Fostering (BAAF)
11 Southwark Street
LONDON SE1 1RQ
Tel: 071 407 8800

For information about adoption and fostering.

British Pregnancy Advisory Service (BPAS)
Austy Manor
Wootton Wawen
SOLIHULL
West Midlands B95 6BX
Tel: 05642 3225

A national network of clinics offering counselling, pregnancy testing and abortion. Ring the telephone number above to find the BPAS clinic nearest to you (or look it up under 'Family planning' or 'Pregnancy' in the Yellow Pages).

Brook Advisory Centres
233 Tottenham Court Road
LONDON W1P 9AE
Tel: 071 580 2991

A network of centres offering advice, help and information to young people (under 26) on personal relationships, contraception, pregnancy and abortion. They also do pregnancy tests. Many of the services are free. Ring the telephone number above to find the Brook Advisory Centre nearest to you. If there is a centre near you, the telephone number might also be in the Yellow Pages under 'Pregnancy'.

Childline
Freepost 1111
LONDON N1 0BR
Tel: 0800 1111

A free telephone counselling service for young people in trouble or danger. You can contact Childline if you are being, or have been, sexually abused.

Equal Opportunities Commission
Overseas House
Quay Street
MANCHESTER M3 3HN
Tel: 061 833 9244

Ring the telephone number above for advice if you are being sexually harassed or sexually discriminated against.

Family Planning Association (FPA)
27-35 Mortimer Street
LONDON W1N 7RJ
Tel: 071 636 7866

Ring the telephone number above to find the family planning clinic nearest to you (or look it up under 'Family planning' in the Yellow Pages). The FPA also runs a free information service and produces free leaflets on contraception.

Friend
Tel: 071 837 3337 (London Friend)

A national advice and counselling service for anyone who is, or thinks they might be, gay. Ring the telephone number above (between 7.30pm and 10.30pm) to find out if there is a Friend branch near you.

Health Education Authority (HEA)
Information Service
c/o Health Promotion Information Centre
Hamilton House
Mabledon Place
LONDON WC1H 9TX
Tel: 071 383 3833

Ring the telephone number above and ask for the Information Service. They can tell you the address of your nearest Health Promotion Unit where you can get free HEA leaflets on many aspects of health education.

Herpes Helpline
Tel: 071 609 9061

A telephone helpline offering advice and information about herpes.

Imperial Cancer Research Fund
PO Box 123
Lincoln's Inn Fields
LONDON WC2A 3PX
Tel: 071 242 0200

Ring the telephone number above for a leaflet on breast self-examination.

Lesbian Line
Tel: 071 251 6911 (London Lesbian Line)

A national advice and counselling service for anyone who is, or thinks they might be, a lesbian. Ring the telephone number above to find out if there is a Lesbian Line near you.

McCormack Ltd (TSE)
Church House
Church Square
LEIGHTON BUZZARD
Bedfordshire LU7 7AE
Tel: 0525 851313

Ring the telephone number above for a leaflet on testicular self-examination.

National AIDS Helpline
Tel: 0800 567123

A national service offering free and confidential advice and information about HIV and AIDS – 24 hours a day, seven days a week. If you are deaf or hard of hearing, you can ring Minicom on 0800 521361 every day from 10am to 10pm. The National AIDS Helpline is also staffed with people who speak:

● Bengali, Gujarati, Hindi, Punjabi, Urdu and English on Wednesdays between 6pm and 10pm.
  Ring 0800 282445.
● Chinese (Cantonese) and English on Tuesdays between 6pm and 10pm.
  Ring 0800 282446.
● Arabic and English on Wednesdays between 6pm and 10pm.
  Ring 0800 282447.

There is an answerphone service in these languages at other times. Leaflets in all the above languages are available.

National Association of Young People's Counselling and Advisory Services (NAYPCAS)
National Youth Bureau
17-23 Albion Street
LEICESTER LE1 6GD
Tel: 0533 558763

Ring the telephone number above to find out if there is a young people's counselling service near you.

National Council for One Parent Families
255 Kentish Town Road
LONDON NW5 2LX
Tel: 071 267 1361

A national service offering free information packs and booklets for single parents.

National Society for the Prevention of Cruelty to Children (NSPCC) Child Protection Helpline
Tel: 0800 800500

A free 24 hour telephone helpline offering advice and information to young people. You can ring this telephone number if you are being, or have been, sexually abused.

Pregnancy Advisory Service (PAS)
11-13 Charlotte Street
LONDON W1P 1HD
Tel: 071 637 8962

Offers counselling, pregnancy tests and abortion.

Rape Crisis Centre
Tel: 071 837 1600 (London Rape Crisis Centre)

To find out the telephone number of the rape crisis centre near you, you can:

● look under 'Rape' in the telephone book
● ring the London Rape Crisis Centre (the number above)
● ring your local Samaritans (look up 'Samaritans' in the telephone book).

Relate
Herbert Gray College
Little Church Street
RUGBY CV21 3AP
Tel: 0788 573241

A national service offering counselling to people with relationship, marriage or sexual problems. Ring the telephone number above to find the branch of Relate nearest to you (or look it up under 'Relate' or 'Marriage guidance' in the telephone book).

Samaritans
If you are feeling desperate or suicidal, you can ring the Samaritans. You can find the telephone number of your local Samaritans in the telephone book under 'Samaritans' or in the front under 'Useful information'.

The Stillbirth and Neonatal Death Society (SANDS)
28 Portland Place
LONDON W1N 4DE
Tel: 071 436 5881

Offers support to parents whose baby has died at or shortly after birth.

Terrence Higgins Trust
52-54 Grays Inn Road
LONDON WC1X 8JU
Tel: 071 242 1010 (helpline)

A telephone helpline giving advice and information about HIV and AIDS. Open from 3pm to 10pm.